Raising a Moody Child

Raising a Moody Child

HOW TO COPE WITH DEPRESSION AND BIPOLAR DISORDER

Mary A. Fristad, PhD, ABPP
Jill S. Goldberg Arnold, PhD

THE GUILFORD PRESS
New York   London

© 2004 The Guilford Press
A Division of Guilford Publications, Inc.
72 Spring Street, New York, NY 10012
www.guilford.com

Printed in the United States of America

This book is printed on acid-free paper.

Last digit is print number: 9   8   7   6   5   4   3   2   1

The lists of symptoms of disorders found on pages 75, 76, 78, 79, and 82 are reprinted with permission from the *Diagnostic and Statistical Manual of Mental Disorders* (4th ed., text revision) by the American Psychiatric Association (Washington, DC). © 2000 American Psychiatric Association.

Library of Congress Cataloging-in-Publication Data

Fristad, Mary A.
  Raising a moody child: how to cope with depression and bipolar disorder / Mary A. Fristad, Jill S. Goldberg Arnold.
    p.   cm.
  Includes bibliographical references and index.
    ISBN 1-57230-871-0 (pbk.: alk. paper) — ISBN 1-57230-930-X (hard)
    1. Depression in children—Popular works.   2. Manic–depressive illness in children—Popular works.   I. Goldberg Arnold, Jill S.   II. Title.
  RJ506.D4F755 2004
  618.92′ 8527—dc21

                                                        2003010339

To our research and clinical families—
thank you for teaching us valuable lessons.

To our own families—
thank you for your love, support, and encouragement.

Contents

Preface

Parenting a child with a mood disorder—or, for that matter, being the child with a mood disorder—can be lonely, frightening, infuriating, heart wrenching, and overwhelming. Whether your child was diagnosed with depression or bipolar disorder two years ago or two weeks ago, or whether you're not yet sure what's wrong, you may be coming to this book exhausted and frustrated. We hope this book will guide you to new strategies for coping and help you navigate the important pathway to developing a local treatment team to work with you and your child. If your child has not yet been diagnosed, we hope our advice for getting an expert evaluation will make that critical first step productive.

Daily, we work with families, perhaps just like yours, to help parents understand what is going on with their mood-disordered child and to help the child or teenager understand as well. In the following pages we share the ideas, information, and tools that we offer to families every day in clinical practice and research. Our experience in working with hundreds of families has taught us that parents (and children) who believe they can improve their situation *do* improve. If this book can provide you with new hope, ease some of your frustration, and diminish any of the pain of living with a mood disorder, we will be satisfied that this job has been well done.

We were moved to write this book by thirty years of collective experience in working with families dealing with affective disorders. I (M. A. F.) began to read with great excitement in the early 1990s about expressed emotion and psychoeducation—that is, psychiatric patient and family education—first for adults with schizophrenia, then for those with mood disorders. Psychoeducation gave a name to the sort of therapy I had concocted for my work with affectively ill children and their parents in response to the fact that no other existing model in the professional literature seemed sufficient to help families cope with their children's symptoms. Over the next ten years our experience with families attending our therapy sessions, groups, and workshops and graciously completing our many interviews and questionnaires convinced us that psychoeducation—which is a supportive, educational, growth-oriented model of clinical intervention—was the best available means we knew to assist families struggling with difficult symptoms and illnesses. Our goal in writing this book is to share with more families than we could ever hope to meet and work with personally the materials we have developed, together and in collaboration with many other colleagues, over our years of research and clinical work with families.

My work in childhood mood disorders, family therapy, and cognitive-behavioral techniques began essentially at the beginning of my training, in the early 1980s, when research on childhood mood disorders was truly in its infancy. For that beginning, I thank Elizabeth B. Weller, MD, Ronald A. Weller, MD, and the faculty in clinical psychology at the University of Kansas. I began to explore psychoeducation as a therapeutic model for children with my colleague Stephen M. Gavazzi, PhD, in the Department of Family Science at the Ohio State University. Beginning in 1993, Dr. Gavazzi, his graduate students Diane Centolella, LISW, and Julie Law, MA, and I did some early work reviewing the literature and developing questionnaires to use in our studies. We began piloting our interventions with the help of Kitty W. Soldano, PhD, LISW, a clinical social worker in the Ohio State University Division of Child and Adolescent Psychiatry. We tried several formats—a workshop for parents of inpatients, which I studied with the assistance of Mitzi Arnett, and outpatient groups. Based on our early group work, we had the good fortune to be funded by the Ohio Department of Mental Health (ODMH) to conduct a pilot study examining the efficacy of multifamily psychoeducation groups (MFPG) in treating children with mood disorders.

By then it was 1998, and Jill S. Goldberg Arnold, PhD, joined the project as the MFPG postdoctoral study coordinator. Her clinical acumen, commitment to the psychoeducation model (which paralleled her doctoral work in developmental disabilities and her internship experiences working with families of children with attention-deficit/hyperactivity disorder), and compassion for the families we were serving made the project a success. Additionally, we continued to benefit from the clinical wisdom of Dr. Soldano, who generously donated her time to the project when we had limited funding to continue. We also appreciated the efforts of several clinical child psychology doctoral students at Ohio State—Kara Fitzpatrick Bijot, MA, Julie Cerel, MA, and Amy Shaver, MA, in particular—whose time and effort allowed us to assess children progressing through the study.

When our study ended, Dr. Goldberg Arnold joined the Ohio State University clinical faculty and provided inpatient and outpatient assessment and therapy services within the Division of Child and Adolescent Psychiatry. In doing so, Dr. Goldberg Arnold was able to further develop and refine many of the child therapy exercises you will see in this book.

We were grateful to receive funding in 2001 from the National Institute of Mental Health to study more thoroughly the efficacy of MFPG in treating children with mood disorders. Because of that, we were able to expand our staff to include Barbara Mackinaw Koons, PhD, the new MFPG postdoctoral study coordinator extraordinaire; Catherine Malkin, PhD, and Dr. Soldano, both of whom are study clinicians; and a cadre of fine graduate students—Kristen Holderle, MA, Dory Phillips Sisson, MA, and Kate Davies Smith, MA—whose energy has helped ensure our current study's success. We have enrolled a majority of the 165 families for this study to date, and you will hear their voices as you peruse the pages of this book.

Most recently, ODMH has again provided pilot funding for a further extension of our work: to study the efficacy of "individual family psychoeducation," or IFP, with twenty families of children ages eight to eleven, all of whom have bipolar disorder. Because of this, Nicholas Lofthouse, PhD, recently joined our staff as the IFP postdoctoral study coordinator, delighting us (and our families) with his British accent and strong commitment to this intervention model.

We continue to appreciate the support received both from the Ohio State University Department of Psychiatry, which provides us with fine space to conduct our clinical research and excellent clinical colleagues and staff, and the Department of Psychology, whose clinical child psychology graduate students and countless advanced undergraduate students continue to impart energy to the project as they join us for practicum and independent study experience.

Although Dr. Goldberg Arnold's family commitments required a move out of state one year ago, it was this move that ultimately freed up enough of her time for us to begin this book together—once again proving the adage that every cloud has a silver lining. Dr. Soldano has continued to be a positive force in this process, as she has carefully edited and

reedited every chapter of the book. We also have had the distinct plea-
sure of working with Kitty Moore and Chris Benton of The Guilford
Press, two fine editors whose knowledge of children's mental health and
family functioning and superb wordsmithery cannot be overstated, to
develop what families who have a child with a mood disorder have been
begging us for—a book to guide them through the murky waters of diagnosis, treatment, and recovery.

In closing, we would be remiss not to note our most important
sources of support—our faith and our families. Our spouses, Joe Fiala
and Moore Arnold, took care of our children, Elise and Peter Fiala and
Aidan and Brendan Arnold, so we could write; our families of origin set
us on this course initially; and our children provided us with a constant
source of inspiration and demonstration of the resiliency and wonder-
ment of childhood.

Part I

Understanding Your Child's Problems

1 | Difficult, Temperamental, Impossible

THE CHALLENGE OF RAISING A MOODY CHILD

Kevin is ten. Although the past ten years have been mostly happy and uneventful, his parents say Kevin has always had a hard time handling disappointments and unexpected events. They've learned to warn him about schedule changes to avoid brief, but sometimes explosive, tantrums. The entire family has gotten used to tiptoeing around Kevin whenever things don't go his way.

Academic success has usually come easily to Kevin, although he has always worried a lot about doing well. Kevin tends to be a worrier in general. His parents have learned to keep the television off during the early evening news so that Keving won't worry about things he hears on the broadcast and have trouble falling asleep. He has lots of good friends at school, in the neighborhood, and on his sports teams.

Starting a couple of months ago, Kevin's parents, Bob and Cindy, noticed that their strategies for helping Kevin cope with changes and disappointments (such as giving him advance warning and providing lots of time and space) have not been enough. He cries easily at the slightest disappointment and has been having more frequent and longer tantrums in response to things not going his way. Although he typically enjoys playing games and spending time with the family, lately they have needed to coax him out of his room during the evenings to join the family in watching a movie or playing a favorite game. He has been complaining about stomachaches almost daily. His teacher sent a note home because she was worried about him; her previously eager and efficient student had not been finishing his work. Kevin's parents have tried asking him what's wrong—whether he feels sick, or whether something happened at school or with one of his friends—but he just grunts and seems to be irritated by the questions.

Over the past couple of weeks, Kevin has gone from staying by himself in his room and mumbling sullenly to snapping at everyone, from Mom and Dad to his eight-year-old sister, Abby, and even his beloved dog, Max, who has slept with Kevin since Max was a puppy. One morning when Max jumped up on Kevin to greet him, Cindy was shocked when Kevin pushed Max away and cursed at him.

Kevin has also begun isolating himself on weekends, reluctant to go to baseball practices and games that formerly he had considered the best parts of his week. He also started turning down invitations to play with his friends. Kevin has started worrying so much about doing well at school that he recently begged his mother to let him stay home—he was convinced that he would fail his social studies quiz if he went to school that day.

Bob and Cindy feel paralyzed. For the last couple of months they have tried everything they could think of, from reading the latest self-help books and magazine articles to doing Internet searches, taking a parenting course through their church, and comparing notes with relatives and friends who have kids. Nothing has helped. In fact, things just seem to be getting worse. Bob was distraught when Abby began complaining that her parents favored her big brother over her. Cindy secretly worries that the family tension will cause her husband, who has not touched alcohol in five years, to begin drinking again—a problem that she does not want to recur.

Kevin's parents have always thought of Kevin as "moody," but they're starting to realize that this seemingly benign term that everyone seems to use does not fully capture what they and their son are experiencing. What could they have done to make Kevin so unhappy? What's really wrong with Kevin?

Feeling at the end of her rope, Cindy made an appointment with Kevin's pediatrician, who ruled out medical problems and referred them to a psychologist. The psychologist did a thorough evaluation and diagnosed Kevin with depression. Knowing what was really wrong was a considerable relief for Bob, Cindy, and even Kevin. Kevin wasn't just "moody," and his parents were neither incompetent nor cruel. Like hundreds of thousands of other American children today, Kevin is depressed. Now he is taking Zoloft, an antidepressant, and attending a combination of individual and family therapy focused on helping Kevin and his parents understand depression, how to manage its symptoms, and how to work together to combat the illness. Things are starting to get better.

Kevin has depression, a mental illness. Reading this book will help you get comfortable with the term *mental illness* and recognize that mood disorders are treatable illnesses. The more comfortable you are with using this and other technical words we introduce in this book, the more you will be able to conquer stigma and to be the best advocate possible for your child.

But what are mood disorders? When we refer to mood disorders, we are talking about two sets of related illnesses: depressive disorders and bipolar disorders. Depressive disorders involve a sad or irritable mood that may last anywhere from a couple of weeks to several years. Bipolar disorders involve alternations between depression and mania, an extremely high mood that can be angry or euphoric. Switches between mania and depression can occur infrequently (e.g., one manic episode during a two-year period) or extremely frequently (e.g., multiple cycles from manic to depressed during a single day). We describe the different depressive and bipolar illnesses in detail in Chapter 2.

Treatment for mood disorders is not, unfortunately, always as straightforward as in Kevin's case. Mood disorders in children are complicated problems. They are not easy to diagnose, in part because the symptoms that children display can look so different from those of adults with mood disorders. For example, children with depression are more often cranky and irritable, whereas adults tend to be melancholy or sad. Adults with bipolar disorder more often experience discrete periods of mania lasting for two to three weeks, followed by a period of depression that might last for several months, whereas children more frequently cycle several times each day between rage, euphoria, and desperate sadness. In addition, in many cases, it can be very difficult to make a diagnosis because the illness is still in the process of developing when an evaluation is completed. For example, if Kevin had been seen three months earlier, when he was struggling to handle changes and disappointments but was generally doing fairly well, depression would not have been an accurate diagnosis. Also, children with mood disorders often have accompanying problems, such as anxiety and behavioral disorders. Kevin is a good example. In addition to depression, he becomes overly anxious and worries excessively about his school performance, as well as about problems and situations that are unrelated to him (such as news items).

Even with treatment, life with a mood-disordered child can feel like a constant challenge—they can be difficult to get along with, seem "impossible" to handle, and generally wreak havoc with domestic tranquility. Their unstable emotional states can disrupt their schoolwork, their friendships, and their sibling bonds. They often need a lot of help to get along in the world, even when they are receiving good treatment.

Thirteen-year-old Caitlyn "never seems happy," according to her parents, and this emotional state is damaging every facet of her life—from her increasingly hostile relationship with her brother to alienation from her classmates (who mock her "Goth" outfits and her matching attitude). Out-and-out exhaustion has started to make her loving parents feel more and more distant from their daughter.

Tanisha, age fifteen, is so sad that she has difficulty speaking above a whisper and getting out of bed. She spends a lot of time crying and can't even pick up the clarinet that she plays with virtuoso skills. The former A student can't complete even short reading assignments. Though she feels guilty for feeling so sad despite what she calls a "great life," Tanisha lashes out in anger or irritation at her parents' constant attempts to comfort her. Her parents are feeling increasingly powerless and helpless.

Six-year-old Jeremiah's parents describe him as "Dr. Jekyll and Mr. Hyde" and then ruefully correct themselves: "He's more like Mr. Hyde and Mr. Hyde," alternating between restless, agitated harangues punctuated by outbursts of rage and slumps of hopelessness and profound sorrow. Their little boy has hit, kicked, and thrown things at his parents, and he has alarmed them several times by gyrating his hips provocatively toward his mother while telling her that he wants to "kiss with you, like in the movies."

Eleven-year-old Anya has shocked family and visitors to her house, running through the house naked, shifting in an instant from hysterical giggling to sobbing, and announcing to everyone who will listen that she can run faster than the cars on the street (and that she has done so) and that she can get 100 percent on all her tests because she can read her teacher's mind.

If any of the children we have described sound at all like your child, you are probably well acquainted with the term *moody*. You have probably felt lost, confused, powerless, and at times hopeless. The many hurdles you have encountered, some of which have seemed insurmountable, have probably overwhelmed you at times. Feeling blamed for your child's problems is exceedingly painful, yet you see blame in the eyes of family members, as well as strangers in the grocery store. Chances are you've felt anger—at your child, yourself, your spouse, your family pet, the person in the car in front of you, or God. The anxiety of not knowing where to turn and not knowing how to help your child can be almost unbearable.

If the children we've described and the feelings of confusion, powerlessness, and hopelessness sound familiar, this book is for you. You may be concerned about your child's behavior, unsure how to make sense out of what doesn't seem "right" to you, and worried about how to *make* it right. If you're wondering where to turn and don't know how to begin, or if you're getting conflicting advice, this book will help you understand what childhood mood disorders are all about—what they look like, how professionals diagnose and treat them, what you need to know about working with your child's school, and how you can manage better at home. In short, we hope that reading this book will help you become a better consumer of mental health care and will empower you to help your son or daughter and your family. Let's begin by replacing some "mood myths" with facts.

Facts versus Myths: Clearing Up the Misconceptions That Keep Moody Kids from Getting Help

Mood disorders in children—depression and bipolar disorder—are widespread, yet they frequently go undiagnosed and are significantly undertreated. Only about one-fourth of the nineteen million American adults with depression seek help. The statistics for children are worse. Additionally, a startling number of teenagers and children with depression are either undiagnosed or misdiagnosed or do not have access to treatment. The failure to identify and treat bipolar disorder in youth is also a significant problem. In a study of the frequency of bipolar disorder in adolescents by Peter Lewinsohn and his colleagues at the Oregon Research Institute, less than half of the teens with bipolar disorder had received any treatment. Current estimates suggest that approximately one-half of 1 percent of all children have bipolar disorder, and we know that one-fourth to one-half of children and adolescents with depression will develop bipolar disorder.

Depression is among the most common of psychiatric disorders, with 10 to 25 percent of women and 5 to 12 percent of men experiencing depression at some point in their lifetimes. At any point in time, conservative estimates reveal that approximately 6 percent of adolescents and 2 percent of preadolescent children are depressed. Depression occurs among people of all ages, income levels, ethnic groups, and cultures (even animals can get depressed). Bipolar spectrum disorders (we define the different types of bipolar disorder in Chapter 2) occur in 3 to 6 percent of the population and occur at equal rates among men and women. Bipolar disorder also occurs in about 1 percent of older adolescents. Approximately 5 percent of older adolescents have enough manic symptoms to cause problems, although not enough to be diagnosed with the full-blown disorder. Prior to adolescence, the rates of bipolar disorder are lower, although Janet Wozniak and Joseph Biederman and their colleagues at Massachusetts General Hospital have found that up to 16 percent of children seen in psychiatric clinics have bipolar disorder. These figures translate as up to 1.8 million teenagers and 600,000 children with depression *at any point in time* and at least 300,000 teenagers and unknown numbers of children with bipolar disorder.[1]

For hundreds of thousands of mood-disordered children and their families, the costs—monetary and otherwise—associated with these disorders are significant. For children, the social price is sky high. If a child is irritable, lacks energy, or behaves unpredictably, other children may dislike her, avoid her, or just ignore her, which leads to many lost play opportunities. Over time these lost opportunities result in the child's falling further behind socially and becoming more and more lonely. Treatment can be expensive and can result in major financial strains for families; even for families with good health care coverage, co-payments for treatment and medication costs can add up quickly. Disagreement between parents about what treatments are necessary or how to discipline their challenging child can lead to marital discord. Tension created by trying to avoid the next crisis can lead to strained relationships and to siblings' feeling that their needs are secondary. Unpredictable or disruptive behavior such as the behavior exhibited by Anya can result in isolation, as the family avoids social gatherings with family and friends for fear of embarrassment.

---

[1] Calculated using 1990 census data and based on data suggesting that 6 percent of adolescents are depressed, 2 percent of children are depressed, and 1 percent of adolescents have bipolar disorder.

This raises an important question: If childhood mood disorders are so widespread and their impact so great, why don't more people seek help? In addition to the complex nature of childhood mood disorders, these disorders are surrounded by many misconceptions that further impede access to treatment.

One primary misconception is that children do not get depressed. Children have no big cares and concerns as adults do, so what could possibly bother them to such a degree that they would get depressed, right? *Wrong!* Mood disorders in children have been recognized only recently—depression beginning in the 1970s and 1980s and bipolar disorder in the mid-1980s. The misconception that mental illnesses are always caused by psychological or environmental factors perpetuated the belief that children could not become depressed or manic. As the understanding of the role of biology, especially genetics, became better understood, childhood mood disorders have been recognized, studied, and treated.

Another myth is the belief that depression will go away quickly and on its own. However, a single episode can last from seven to nine months, an entire school year. And 40 percent of children who have had a single depressive episode will have another one within two years, 70 percent within five years. A single episode can wreak havoc with the life of a child and his family. Repeated episodes result in exponentially more damage. Just to make things more complicated, the course of depression and bipolar disorders is often unpredictable. Treatment can be helpful in reducing the frequency and severity of episodes, but families need to be on the lookout for signs of recurrence. It is clear that symptoms tend to worsen over time, making early and effective treatment particularly important.

The myth that "everybody gets that way" is common. Although we all have our good days and bad days, we don't all reach clinical highs and lows as a response to positive and negative life events. In Chapter 2, we provide a pictorial view of the different patterns mood disorders can take—that picture gives some perspective on the difference between normal variations in mood and the distinctly unhealthy vacillations that children with mood disorders experience. Take ten-year-old Kevin as an example. It is typical for kids to get upset in response to disappointment, but Kevin struggles excessively to recover and is unable to handle even minor disappointments. All kids can be silly and sometimes even claim superpowers as part of their play, but Anya's hysterical giggling punctuated by sobbing and her outlandish claims are outside the bounds of normal childhood behavior.

Yet another myth is the belief that those with depression should "just snap out of it." No one would ever dream of telling a child with strep throat or an ear infection to just "snap out" of the discomfort he or she was experiencing. Instead, children who are sick are taken to the doctor and prescribed treatment. Mood disorders are also illnesses and require specialized treatment. In some cases the treatment will involve medication. However, finding the optimal medication or combination of medications for a particular set of mood symptoms is not always easy. In many cases, medication will help, but only partially. Therapy is also an important part of treatment for mood disorders. Therapy comes in many variations; deciding whom to see and what to try can be complicated. In Part II of this book we discuss the specifics of different types of treatment and help you begin to develop a road map for accessing the treatment your child needs.

One of the most damaging myths is that getting treatment is a sign of weakness or failure. Many adults avoid getting treatment for themselves because they fear appearing weak. This is also true of teenagers or older children, who feel that they should be able to "pull it together" themselves. Parents sometimes avoid seeking treatment for their children for fear they will be seen as having failed in parenting. This myth leads many to delay seeking treatment or, worse yet, not to seek help at all.

Another myth is that all adolescents are moody and that, therefore, there is no need to focus attention on their condition. Although teenagers, in particular, have their ups and downs as they develop their own personas, "normal" fluctuations in mood are less frequent, less intense, and less long lasting than the types of mood changes we see in clinical depression or bipolar disorder. For example, at first glance Caitlyn might seem like a normal teenager. She is "making a statement" with the way she dresses, although her statement is alienating her from many of her peers. She spends a lot of time in her own room, but she has shut herself off completely from her family and is irritable and rude in her interactions at home. Most important, she never seems happy. Healthy teenagers find enjoyment: They might not look forward to family game night with eagerness, but there should be signs that they are having fun at least some of the time. It's not uncommon for teenagers to pare down their interests and activities and to begin to pursue a few interests at a greater level of depth. Dropping out of all or most activities and seeming uninterested in anything is not part of adolescence.

Finally, mood-impaired children and adolescents are often considered "bad" or "lazy" because of their frequently disruptive, surly, or even enraged behavior, as well as their lethargy, lack of interest, and difficulty concentrating. These pejorative interpretations of symptoms contribute to negative interactions between them and their parents, teachers, and others. When symptoms are perceived to be negative traits rather than signs of significant problems and a need for help, a major barrier to seeking treatment is erected.

What Can I Expect to Gain from Reading This Book?

In addition to the myths about mood disorders that pervade our society, parents who are seeking help for a child with any kind of psychological problem run into some common roadblocks along the way. The very first one, to which few parents seem impervious, is self-blame. Self-blame is all too common among parents of children with mood disorders. Parents of children with mood disorders frequently ruminate over what they have done to make their child so unhappy or to have provoked such interminably long and severe tantrums. Tanisha's parents, like many parents of depressed children, ask themselves what they have done wrong, and six-year-old Jeremiah's parents have frequently wondered how they allowed his behavior to get so out of control. The reality is that neither Tanisha's nor Jeremiah's parents caused their children's problems. Both Jeremiah and Tanisha have biological illnesses, their parents are in no way to blame. Unfortunately, self-blame only increases the pain that parents face.

The corollary to self-blame is blaming each other. Caitlyn's father has accused his wife of catering to her too much, whereas Caitlyn's mother feels that her husband has been too hard on Caitlyn and has alienated her. Blaming each other only increases tension, making it more difficult to get treatment and, ultimately, to solve the problem of managing symptoms.

Beyond self-blame there are some practical challenges that many families face. Insurance coverage is often limited to only a few providers within a community, and those providers may not have specific expertise in childhood mood disorders. In addition, good providers often have long waiting lists. It is not uncommon for families to wait two to three months for an initial evaluation. Two or three months (or even one week) can seem like an eternity when your child is having daily rages, is not falling asleep until 1:00 or 2:00 A.M., and is so irritable that having a conversation has become impossible.

The evaluation process can sometimes be frustrating and time-consuming. Childhood mood disorders can be especially difficult to separate from such behavioral problems as poor attention, hyperactivity, impulsivity, and oppositional and defiant behavior. Although many providers are well versed in childhood problems, only a small subset are experts in childhood mood disorders. You may find yourself needing a second opinion following that first evaluation for which you waited so long.

Once you find a provider you trust, and once he or she has completed a thorough evaluation and has made a diagnosis with which you feel comfortable, determining how to proceed can still be a challenge. One question that many parents face is whether or not to medicate. Weighing the pros and cons of medications can be difficult—medications often have side effects, but they may improve quality of life overall. There are also many types of therapy and many different characteristics of therapists. Many different combinations of family members could potentially participate in therapy, ranging from the child alone to the whole family and even including extended family when relevant. Chapters 6 and 7 provide details about negotiating decisions on medications and therapy.

The steps required to get the right help sometimes occur swiftly and smoothly, but often some impediments occur along the way. If you feel unsure of how to proceed, you aren't alone. In this book, we walk you through the steps you need to take to get past these roadblocks and get on your way to helping your child.

The primary goal of this book is to help you find the assistance your child needs. We begin by helping you understand what you're seeing in your child, then we provide you with strategies to manage the challenges and frustrations that come with raising a moody child. Above all, we hope to help you become the best possible advocate for your child. You know your child best, and you spend far more time with your child than anyone else. Thus you are ultimately the most important member of your child's mental health team. With the information and advice in this book, we hope you will gain the confidence to make good decisions for your child, using the recommendations of the professionals on your team.

How Is This Book Organized?

Part I of this book describes mood symptoms and syndromes. You will learn about the evaluation and diagnosis process and about depression and bipolar disorder (manic–depression) in children. You will become familiar with different mood symptoms and how they fit into each diagnostic category. As you read (and as you work with treatment providers) you will be asked about a variety of symptoms that you have noticed in your child. Your treatment providers (and you, as you read) will start to notice particular clusters of symptoms in your child and will begin to label them in psychiatric terms. This is an important early step in getting good treatment. Developing a better overall understanding of mood disorders and a better specific understanding of your child's problem will equip you to find good treatment, reduce sources of conflict, and improve life for your child, yourself, and your family. Part I shows you how to become the best possible consumer of mental health services. Some of the most important decisions you will make for your child will involve choosing the professionals on your treatment team. You'll also learn how to find appropriate services and know what to expect from each of them. Before you can choose among professionals, you need to know what kind to look for, and you need to have an understanding of what to expect.

In Part II you'll learn about the different types of treatments available for children with mood disorders and their families. As you learn about the different medications and types of therapy available, you will come to understand the *biopsychosocial* model of treatment. Mood disorders are biological illnesses and therefore often require biological treatments such as medications. They are also psychological conditions, meaning that they result in problems with thoughts, feelings, and behavior, and therefore children and families typically require some sort of therapy to develop healthier patterns of thinking and behavior that ultimately help improve mood. And children with mood disorders function in a variety of social settings—mostly at home and at school—and therefore often need to have some temporary adjustments made in these settings. You'll learn about the different goals for each type of treatment and about how to complete a cost–benefit analysis to help you choose the appropriate treatment components for your child.

Part III focuses on how you can help your child. You'll learn coping skills for you and your child to use. Some of these skills, such as communication and problem-solving strategies, are good for families in general. We anticipate that you'll find them particularly beneficial as you work together to manage your child's mood symptoms. Information and suggestions on how to work with your school system and how to manage crises are also provided.

Finally, Part IV focuses on how you can help your family. Reading this section will help you recognize and break negative cycles that can occur within families stressed by the presence of a mood disorder. You will learn how to create a balance for your family, how to help siblings, and how to take care of yourself. We hope your journey through this book provides you the support, knowledge, and skill building you need to move forward productively.

2 | What's Wrong with My Child?

In Chapter 1 you met some children who may have sounded very familiar to you. At this point you probably have more questions than answers. Does my child have a mood disorder? What if my child doesn't exactly fit the description of the children I read about in Chapter 1? My child can look so very different at different times of the day and in different settings—is this really a mood disorder?

In this chapter we help you understand what the different types of mood disorders look like in a variety of children so that you can begin to get an idea of whether the behavior you're seeing in your child may be caused by a mood disorder. We don't expect you to diagnose your own child, but rather to gather enough information to decide whether to make an appointment for a thorough evaluation. Identifying mood disorders can be a complicated process, but you can use the same information and the same types of measurements that professionals use to take an objective look at your child. If, after applying those guidelines, you believe your child should be evaluated for a mood disorder, Chapter 4 will guide you through the evaluation process and lay out the precise criteria used to diagnose each mood disorder.

Is It Really a Problem?

When we're worried that something might be wrong with our child, most of us struggle with the question of how bad the problem really is and how urgently the child needs professional help. Protectiveness and love for our child may keep us bouncing between the urge to rush our child to the doctor in a panic and the hope that if we wait just a little longer, the problem will go away. Objectivity can be elusive! We suggest that you use this simple rule: *It's a problem when it's a problem.* By that we mean that problem behaviors are considered mood symptoms if they cause distress, interfere with children's functioning, or both. Ask yourself this question: Do the behaviors cause your child significant problems at home, at school, or with other children? For teenagers who are employed outside the home, is there noticeable impairment in their work setting?

To begin to get an idea of whether your child has a mood disorder, you need to know what mood states are, how clinicians measure them, and how symptoms may cluster together in a child.

Defining Mood States

The first step in determining whether a child has a mood disorder is figuring out which moods occur—sadness, irritability, euphoria, rage? This is a critical step because the kinds of moods your child experiences determine whether she fits into either the depressive or bipolar group of disorders.

Depressive disorders always include one of three cardinal symptoms: sad mood, irritable mood, or loss of interest. In this case, loss of interest doesn't just mean that your child has gotten bored with a previously enjoyed activity (most children change interests as they mature); it means that your child has stopped getting enjoyment out of activities available on a day-to-day basis. When Kaylee comes home from school, she slumps down on the couch, turns down friends who come to the door to ask her to play, and ignores her kitten, which she used to play with every afternoon. She has begun refusing to go to soccer practice, even though she loves her coach and is a very good athlete.

Children with bipolar disorders display a combination of moods that are too low (depression) and too high (mania). Part of what makes diagnosing bipolar disorder so complex is that many different combinations of moods might occur. What you need to look for in your child are extreme moods such as rage and elation or euphoria. Recent research by a leading expert on childhood bipolar disorder, Barbara Geller, and her colleagues at Washington University has shown the occurrence of elated mood to be one of the clearest indicators of bipolar disorder. Because bipolar disorder involves switching back and forth between high and low moods, you may have also noticed sadness and irritability.

Measuring the Problem

Once you've determined which moods your child is experiencing, ask yourself, "How bad is it?" Clinicians use three yardsticks to measure this: how often does the problem occur (frequency), how long does it last (duration), and how bad is it when it happens (severity)?

FREQUENCY

How often do your child's problems occur? All children experience episodic difficulties representative of most depressive and many manic symptoms at some point or another as part of their routine development. But frequent difficulties are an important early clue for clinicians trying to determine how "off" a behavior is. For example, we all have nights when we can't fall asleep. An elementary-age child may be worried about his first "big" math test the next day, a middle schooler could be preoccupied with a note passed to her by her best friend's new boyfriend, or a teenager might be pondering college applications, and all could have some restless nights as a result. Life is like that. Clinicians become concerned when someone can't fall asleep night after night for weeks on end.

Likewise, rages can occur once a week or three times a day. With bipolar disorder, keeping track of the number of cycles between different mood states your child experiences is important. Some children cycle so rapidly that it's difficult to pick out when the changes occur. In these cases parents often describe their children as "constantly cycling." (We discuss cycling later in this chapter.)

DURATION

How much time your child spends feeling sad, irritable, enraged, or elated is also critical to determining the significance of the problem. Constant sadness or irritability are more severe symptoms, as are longer periods of rage or elation. But assessing the duration of symptoms is complicated for children whose moods change frequently—rage episodes may last for only twenty minutes each, but if six rage episodes occur each day separated by periods of profound sadness and periods of

agitated excitement, the overall amount of time of daily mood disturbance is high and thus represents serious mood impairment.

SEVERITY

When a child is evaluated, the severity of the mood symptoms will be ex-
amined carefully and will help determine which diagnosis is most appropriate and how aggressively treatment should be pursued. Just as taco
sauce comes in various strengths—mild, medium, and hot—so can mood
symptoms be rated as mild, moderate, or severe.

In ordinary life, sadness, anger, and happiness all occur on a continuum and match the situation in which they occur. We expect a child to
feel sad when a friend moves away, angry when his younger brother
breaks his favorite toy, or happy when her soccer team wins a tourna-
ment. Does your child's mood seem appropriate in response to the situations he encounters?

To judge the severity of mood symptoms, you also need to know
how the child's current moods compare with her typical moods before
you began noticing any change; or, with a child whose mood has seemed
"off" since birth, how different your child is from other children. Nadya,
ten, has always been bubbly, with an infectious laugh that comes easily
and frequently. But a few months ago her mother noticed that she
seemed more serious. At the time, her parents chalked it up to Nadya's
getting older, but then Nadya began talking a lot about her cat, which
had died several years ago, and her laughter became rarer, her nearly
constant smile sometimes replaced by a sad expression. Over the past
month, Nadya began looking sad most of the time, getting uncharacteris-
tically tearful several times but unable to explain why when asked. Over
the past week, her sadness seemed to escalate even further. Now she
sobs uncontrollably several times a day and appears to be so sad that she
looks like she's in pain. Even her playful kitten and her favorite cartoon
don't bring a smile to her face. Nadya's sadness started out mild, though
it was still a significant change from her typical demeanor; then it progressed to a moderate level of sadness, and finally to a severely impaired
mood.

Irritability can also be mild, moderate, or severe. Fourteen-year-
old Emily is typically easygoing and helpful around the house, but
lately she's been easily irritated—even at the one-year-old cousin she
adores—and grumbles whenever her mother asks her to do the simplest
chore, such as setting the table. Twelve-year-old Evan is lashing out

without provocation—he screamed at his mother when she asked him a question while he was watching TV—and the slightest change in the family's plans can throw him so thoroughly that he just can't recover and ends up isolating himself, missing out on events such as the movie his family went to last week. And the situation has reached a crisis point for ten-year-old Bethany, who is so irritable she can barely tolerate being in the room with anyone else. Everything from her brother sitting down next to her on the couch to her mother asking her what she would like for dinner results in an angry tirade. When things don't go her way, she yells and screams. Last week, when it was her brother's turn to choose a TV show, Bethany got so angry and worked up that she followed her mother around the house arguing her point for the whole length of the show. Emily, Evan, and Bethany illustrate the continuum of irritability. As with sadness, however, keep in mind that severity is a subjective judgment unless it's tied to something measurable, such as a change from the child's typical functioning of the past.

Happiness also falls on a continuum and generally should match the situation in degree and frequency. About three weeks ago, fifteen-year-old Marcia, typically described as calm and serious, started laughing too hard and too long and at the wrong things. She giggled for several minutes when her mother told Marcia that her brother had broken his ankle. Marcia didn't seem to think her behavior was odd, so at first her parents tried not to be concerned. But about a week later Marcia began laughing aloud and uncontrollably in the middle of church, telling her parents that the pastor's sermon had been hilariously funny, even though the rest of the congregation had only chuckled quietly. Later that week, during math class, Marcia began laughing and screaming with excitement after doing a math problem correctly on the board, describing how she had been enlightened and could solve the world's problems. Marcia's mood elevation started out mildly, but its escalating severity was a strong indicator of mania.

Symptom Clustering

As you'll see in Chapter 4, a number of symptoms besides mood are associated with each mood disorder. To make a diagnosis, a certain number of symptoms must be present at the same time. Remember Tanisha from Chapter 1? Her crying, loss of interest in her clarinet, and irritability with her parents, all of which have been occurring for two months, are examples of the cluster of symptoms that indicate depression. Anya, with her speeding around, fast talking, and sleeplessness, is a good example of how manic symptoms might cluster together. Identifying which symptoms occur along with mood disturbance also helps to determine which diagnosis best fits your child.

Is It a Mood Disorder or Some Other Problem?

Your child may seem to have all the signs and symptoms of a mood disorder, but before a clinician will diagnose him or her with a specific disorder, the doctor will need to make sure that the problem isn't caused by something else entirely. The cause of the symptoms is important because it can determine what treatment is appropriate and effective. You need to know that your child's problems are not the result of other medications or illegal drugs, another physical illness, or temporary stressors. For example, some asthma medications can make children irritable. Rather than counting this as a symptom of a mood disorder, we would consider the irritability a side effect of the asthma medicine. If your child experiences side effects from medications for other medical conditions, we recommend that you work with your primary care physician or specialist to determine whether another type of medicine or dosage regimen would effectively manage that illness without causing the unpleasant side effect of irritable mood. Another good example is low iron (anemia), which can result in symptoms that look like depression (e.g., low energy). If your child's low energy is a symptom of a dietary deficiency rather than a mood disorder, it should go away when the anemia is diagnosed and an iron supplement is added to her diet. If thyroid disorders run in your family and if your child appears to have too much or too little energy, have her thyroid level checked. Teenagers (and children) who use marijuana can appear lethargic and unmotivated. If you have any concern that your child might be using illicit substances, talk to his primary care physician about conducting random drug screens.

It is also important to determine whether anything is happening that might be causing your child to behave in particular ways. Children are great barometers of their environment, and they reflect almost anything that's going on around them. If stress is running high because of financial problems, marital tension, an illness in the family, or a personality conflict with a teacher, chances are that your child will reflect those concerns. A child who is experiencing a sad or irritable mood in response to a stressful family or school situation should be diagnosed with an adjustment disorder rather than a mood disorder and provided with appropriate support and therapy.

What Do Mood Disorders Look Like?

Figuring out what moods your child experiences, how severe those moods are, how long they last, how often they happen, and how they cluster with other problems will give you, and later a clinician, a fairly good idea of whether your child has one of the mood disorders, but it won't provide all the necessary information to diagnose or rule out a specific disorder. There are several different depressive disorders and several types of bipolar disorder. Each of the different disorders involves impaired mood, which is the reason these conditions are referred to as mood disorders. The mood impairment may be mild, moderate, or severe and may last only a couple of weeks or may persist for much longer. If your child has a depressive disorder, she experiences a sad or irritable mood, which may take several forms. In a major depressive disorder (MDD) a child's mood is markedly different from "normal," and numerous accompanying symptoms occur. A milder but more chronic low mood is typical of *dysthymic disorder* (DD). We refer to dysthymic disorder as the "low-grade fever" of mood disorders.

Individuals with bipolar disorder Type I (BP I) have moods that shift from depression to mania, whereas those with bipolar disorder Type II (BP II) experience periods of depression cycling with periods of mildly elevated mood called *hypomania*. And those with cyclothymia cycle from mild depression to hypomania. The diagnosis of bipolar disorder not otherwise specified, or BP-NOS, is used to describe individuals who don't fit criteria for any of the specific bipolar disorders but who have clear alterations in mood that include both depressive and manic elements. A large proportion of children with bipolar disorder fall into this category. In particular, children who cycle back and forth between profound sadness, rage, and elation several times each day are often labeled as having BP-NOS.

A Picture Is Worth a Thousand Words

To get a graphic idea of how the mood disorders differ from each other and from a normal mood, look at Figure 1, which illustrates how the major mood disorders appear over time. Panel A shows a normal mood, with the typical ups and downs of daily life. Dysthymic disorder is depicted in Panel B. In this "low grade fever," the mood dips slightly below normal and stays there for a prolonged period of time. Panel C illustrates major depression: the mood dips far below normal, then stays there for a

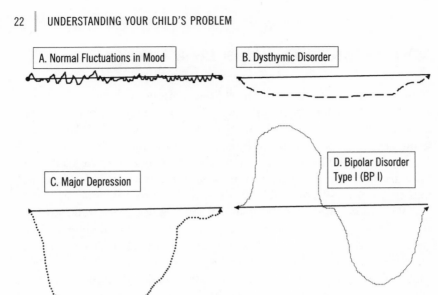

A. Normal Fluctuations in Mood

B. Dysthymic Disorder

C. Major Depression

D. Bipolar Disorder Type I (BP I)

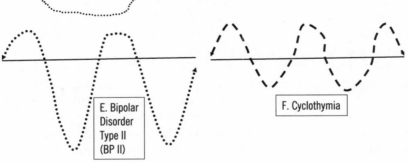

E. Bipolar Disorder Type II (BP II)

F. Cyclothymia

FIGURE 1 The patterns of mood disorders.

significant period of time. In Panel D you see an individual with BP I. This individual experiences an excessively high mood, mania, followed by a period of very low mood, depression. Panel E shows the mood of an individual with BP II, who experiences periods of high mood (referred to as *hypomania* because it is not as high as mania) and periods of depression. And Panel F depicts cyclothymia, with periods of mildly elevated and mildly depressed moods. Figure 2 shows one way in which BP-NOS might appear—with constant cycling between desperate sadness, rage, and euphoria. Whereas this pattern is somewhat uncommon in adults, recent research by Barbara Geller and her colleagues at Washington University has shown that up to 77 percent of children with bipolar disorder exhibit this pattern.

Understanding Cycling

If you have a child who has or may have a mood disorder, it's important that you understand cycling, a primary feature of several mood diagnoses. *Cycling* is the term that describes switches between various degrees of depressed and manic symptoms. The essential feature of bipolar illness is the changing of mood from mania to depression. However, children are much more likely than adults to experience rapid cycling. Barbara Geller and her colleagues have described three different patterns of rapid cycling:

1. Rapid cycling: up to four manic episodes per year
2. Ultrarapid cycling: 5 to 364 manic episodes per year
3. Ultradian or continuous cycling: 365 or more episodes per year, with manic mood (extremely irritable or extremely elated or expansive) occurring for at least four hours per day

When cycling occurs rapidly, as in Figure 2, a child's mood might go from intense sadness to raging anger in just a few minutes. Needless to say, this is very distressing, for both the child and his or her family members, who are not sure how to react from moment to moment. This pat-

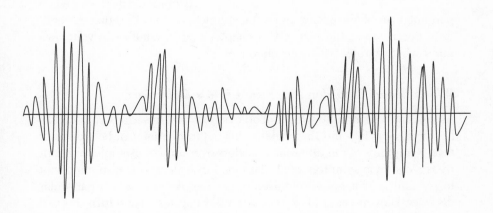

FIGURE 2   Continuous cycling bipolar disorder (diagnosed as BP-NOS).

tern is not actually described in the current diagnostic manual and therefore is often referred to as bipolar disorder not otherwise specified (BP-NOS). With moods changing so frequently, it is easy to see how hard it must be for a parent to come up with a firm opinion about whether the child has a depressive or bipolar disorder. The task becomes even tougher when you factor in what is termed a *mixed state* presentation, described in greater detail later. In a mixed state, symptoms of depression and mania occur at the same time. Diagnosticians will do their best to distinguish among mood disorders in children by paying particularly close attention to your descriptions of your child's mood, how your child's symptoms cluster, and when

WHAT IF MY CHILD DOESN'T FIT THE PICTURE FOR A SPECIFIC MOOD DISORDER?

If your child doesn't quite fit the picture of one particular mood disorder from what you've read so far, don't despair. It doesn't mean that you won't be able to get help. It's not uncommon for kids to have mood disorder symptoms without conforming to a precise diagnosis, because children are continuously developing and their symptoms may still be evolving. Additionally, diagnostic criteria were written based on observations of adults with mood disorders. Children are not miniature adults, and their symptoms can sometimes look different from those of adults. Adults with bipolar disorder, for example, tend to have far fewer cycles between mania and depression than do children. A sharp diagnostician will know this and will diagnose bipolar disorder in children when appropriate. But even if your child's doctor doesn't want to diagnose a particular disorder, there are treatments available that can help the child lead a happier, more successful life. (See Part II of this book for more information.)

particular problems began. In the meantime, you may find that the children described in the rest of this chapter help crystallize in your own mind what's wrong with your child.

Which Mood Disorder Fits Your Child's Behavior?

As you try to determine which mood disorder best describes your child's behavior, bear in mind that making this determination can be a difficult task. Symptoms of the different disorders overlap. For example, irritability is a common symptom of all the mood disorders. It is also important to remember that not all children have every symptom of a particular disorder. Eleven-year-old Mark is sad every day, tosses and turns for two hours before finally falling asleep at night, and has trouble mustering enough energy to get dressed in the morning or to play a game with his brother. Ten-year-old Maria snaps at everyone in the family throughout the day, is so restless that she can't sit still during school, and has a terrible time waking up each morning. These two children have different subsets of depressive symptoms. However, Maria also has periods during which she becomes giddy and her energy level skyrockets. Last week her mother was at a loss as to what to do when she went into Maria's room and found her laughing while using way too much of her mother's makeup, trying on every outfit in her closet, and drawing pictures of all of the dresses she was going to make with her mother's sewing machine. Different snapshots of symptoms can point toward different disorders; this can make it very difficult to differentiate between disorders, even for professionals.

Perhaps the most important distinction to make is whether a child has a depressive or a bipolar spectrum disorder. Treatments differ between these two categories of illness. In some cases, the wrong diagnosis may lead to a treatment that exacerbates the child's existing problems. For example, antidepressants when prescribed alone can worsen manic symptoms. In addition to guiding treatment, knowing your child's diagnosis helps you develop realistic expectations for treatment and will help you as you develop a plan to manage your child's symptoms.

When Did the Problems Start?

As you navigate through the process of finding the appropriate diagnosis for your child, you will probably be asked when the problems began. This question is important because the duration of symptoms may help to determine the diagnosis. It is also important because when and how your child's symptoms started may significantly affect how his symptoms progress. Six-year-old Jeremiah's symptoms started so early that his parents have a hard time pinpointing their appearance—it seems as though the problems have always been there in one form or another. On the other hand, sixteen-year-old Ruth had always been an A student, had lots of friends, and had been involved in a variety of school activities. All of a sudden, one week during her junior year, her thoughts began racing, she began talking about her power to change the world and make everyone follow her, she began staying up most of the night writing her "manifesto," and her mood seemed to be flying high. Jeremiah has the disadvantage of never having experienced normal development. Ruth has a strong base to work from but experiences the pain of knowing what life was like when she was free of a mood disorder. Her glass is both half empty and half full. Your management strategies may need to differ based on whether your child's mood disorder came on suddenly without any previous problems or whether the mood symptoms came on gradually and were preceded by other problems (e.g., behavioral problems).

Major Depressive Disorder

Luis is seven. Last year he was diagnosed with attention-deficit/hyperactivity disorder (ADHD) and responded well to treatment with a stimulant medication. Over the past month or so, Luis has begun showing signs of mood problems for the first time. He has become clingy. At a recent family get-together, Luis spent the entire evening curled up on his grandmother's lap, despite repeated attempts by his cousins to get him to come play. When his mother takes the children to the playground, he sits with his mother on the bench rather than partaking in his usual exuberant climbing. His teacher called home concerned because Luis had begun crying on the playground for no clear reason twice over the past two weeks—an unusual event for Luis, who usually looks forward to recess.

Recently Luis has seemed tired, and he has started to complain about being bored. When his mother suggests that he build with his Legos or work on his model car, he just shrugs his shoulders and wanders back to his room. He has also been resisting going to baseball practice, whereas previously Luis would beg to wear his baseball uniform to school every day. At night he has been finding many excuses to delay going to bed. When Luis's parents have gone to check on him before going to bed themselves, they have found him still awake. A few times, Luis's mother has heard noises, gone downstairs, and found him watching TV at 1:00 or 2:00 A.M. Despite his mother making his favorite meals and even enticing him with sugar-coated cereal, Luis has been uninterested in eating, so much so that his pants have started to get loose. His parents were particularly concerned when two of his friends came by after school to ask him to play and he turned them down.

A child with major depressive disorder (MDD) may be very sad or very irritable (or both at the same or different times) or may demonstrate a loss of interest in previously enjoyable activities. Because typically developing children also have bad days and may experience several days in a row of being sad or irritable in response to an unpleasant event, it's important to know that a child will not be diagnosed with major depressive disorder unless the symptoms have persisted for at least a couple of weeks.

Maybe your child doesn't behave exactly like Luis. To get an impression of whether he or she may have major depressive disorder, answer these questions:

Does your child:

▥ Have periods of sadness daily?

Luis comes home from school looking miserable every day. He cries at the drop of a hat, and smiles have become very infrequent, which is in stark contrast to his usually good sense of humor and frequent smiles.

▥ Have daily periods of irritability or anger that last most of the day?

Luis is very quick to anger, especially in the afternoons and evenings. He gets angry at his younger sister (age three) for things that would not have angered him before, such as requesting that he play with her. He has even begun to get angry at the family dog for things such as bringing his favorite ball and trying to get Luis to play.

Twelve-year-old Sharon is so irritable that her parents have begun to feel they can never say the right thing. Yesterday she jumped down her mother's throat for complimenting her outfit. She has accused her family of picking on her, but they feel like they have bent over backward to make things better for her.

▥ Seem to have lost interest or complain of boredom?

After school, Luis complains that he has nothing to do. His mother makes suggestions, such as riding his bike or scooter, finding a friend to play catch with, or jumping on the trampoline, all favorite activities in the past. He shows no interest. At first, his mother thought that maybe he had just gotten tired of his old activities. As his birthday was soon approaching, she took him to the toy store to point out items he might like as presents. He walked around the toy store looking miserable and just shrugged whenever she pointed out something she thought he might like.

▥ Seem to have stopped enjoying previously fun activities?

Luis is a good athlete and has typically enjoyed playing sports such as soccer and baseball. He recently told his mother that he wanted to quit playing soccer and that he does not want to be in Boy Scouts anymore.

Sharon complains constantly that she is bored. She had looked forward all summer to trying out for her middle school's basketball team. By the time tryouts came up in the fall, she wouldn't go. Sharon told her parents that she wants to quit taking piano lessons. They insisted that she finish out the year but are beginning to regret pushing the issue because she refuses to practice. Sharon spends most of her time either sitting and watching TV, surfing the Web, or listening to CDs in her room. When friends call, she makes excuses not to get together. Her parents initially saw Sharon's behavior as part of her becoming an adolescent. It wasn't until Sharon's aunt raised the question of depression that her parents became concerned about her mood.

■ Have trouble falling asleep at night?

Luis has begun having greater and greater difficulty getting up in the morning for school despite a consistent 8:30 P.M. bedtime. His mother started checking on him at night even though he was quiet. Only then did she realize that Luis was not falling asleep until 10:00 or 11:00 P.M. He used to fall asleep within ten minutes after lying down in his bed.

Some children will show their sleeplessness by falling asleep at any moment, looking groggy during the day, or requiring caffeinated beverages (usually sodas) to stay awake throughout their school day.

■ Wake up in the middle of the night and have trouble getting back to sleep?

Several times during the past month, Luis's parents have heard noises in the house and have found Luis in the living room watching TV at 1:00 or 2:00 A.M.

Middle-of-the-night wakings also may result in children asking to get into bed with parents. Some children do not get out of bed at all but spend a fair amount of time tossing and turning. By the same token, parents are often unaware of sleep problems. This situation underscores the importance of interviewing both parents and children when conducting an evaluation.

■ Wake up very early in the morning?

On other occasions, Luis has gone into his parents' room at 4:30 or 5:00 A.M. and told them that he could not sleep any longer. He is particularly tired and cranky on these days.

■ Sleep too much?

Luis's mother talked to her sister, whose twelve-year-old son Eduardo has been diagnosed with depression. Eduardo goes to bed at

9:30 P.M. and has a terrible time getting up by 7:30 A.M. to get ready for school. On the weekends, he sleeps until 1:00 or 2:00 P.M. after going to bed by 10:00 P.M.

■ Eat too much as a result of being sad, irritable, or anxious?

Eduardo has gained ten pounds (but has not grown in height) over the past three months and is beginning to look overweight. He craves carbohydrates and will eat entire packages of chips or crackers if not carefully supervised. However, Eduardo is a picky eater and has little interest in what his mother prepares for meals.

■ Eat too little as a result of being sad, irritable, or anxious?

Over the past month, Luis's clothes have gotten looser, and he has mostly pushed the food around on his plate, even his favorites. When asked, Luis tells his mother that he just isn't hungry. Some children don't lose weight but stop eating all but a few foods that they really like, or they don't gain weight as expected over a sustained period of time.

■ Have trouble concentrating?

Despite the fact that Luis takes his Adderall consistently, Luis's teacher recently sent a note home because Luis seemed to be having difficulty staying on task.

Tanisha has always been a good student. As she became increasingly depressed, however, it became harder for her to stay focused on what she was hearing at school. Her teachers never suspected a problem because Tanisha had always been quiet and appeared attentive. Her parents were unaware of the problem until she started crying inconsolably after trying unsuccessfully to complete a short reading assignment for history, her favorite class.

Although Sharon's standardized test scores have been consistently high, her grades have typically been average to mediocre. The one exception is math, in which Sharon has always excelled and typically gotten A's. She recently failed a math test. When her math teacher asked Sharon if anything was wrong, she burst into tears and ran out of his classroom.

Changes in concentration as the result of a mood disorder are sometimes difficult to separate from co-occurring problems (e.g., ADHD) and in some cases may be hard to spot. The key is to note any changes in your child's concentration or school performance, as declining grades may be the first indicator of concentration difficulties.

▓ Seem tired despite sleeping enough?

Despite getting twelve or more hours of sleep per night, Eduardo has seemed tired during the day. Each day when he comes home from school, Eduardo lies down on the couch to watch TV and often falls asleep.

▓ Seem restless?

At times, Luis can't seem to sit still. He will turn the TV on, then walk in circles around the room, barely seeming to pay attention to the show. He has begun chewing on the ends of his shirt collars and cuffs. Since Luis was diagnosed with ADHD, his parents have gotten used to his generally high level of motor activity, especially as his medication wears off. However, whereas his "ADHD activity" appears more "busy-like," what Luis's parents are noticing now appears more like nervous energy.

▓ Seem lethargic?

Over the past month, Eduardo has been much less active than usual. It seems to take him a long time to do anything. Eduardo's teacher has reported to his parents that he looks "droopy" during the school day.

In some cases, the same child will seem slow and lethargic at some times and restless and agitated at other times. As with concentration, it is important to note *changes* in activity level: A typically active child becoming slow and lethargic or a typically calm child becoming restless and agitated is an indicator that something is wrong.

▓ Feel worthless?

When his mother tried to figure out why Luis wanted to quit playing soccer and participating in Boy Scouts, he said, "I can't play anyway," and "No one in my den likes me."

▓ Feel excessively guilty?

Luis recently became tearful after recalling a fight he had with his younger sister, during which he pushed her away from one of his toys that he didn't want her to touch. His sister wasn't injured, and the fight had occurred several months ago.

Tanisha is very concerned that she's causing problems for her family. She berates herself for "being a burden" and for not being grateful for what she has. Her guilt over burdening her family sometimes precipitates crying spells.

▦ Express suicidal or morbid thoughts?

It became clear to Luis's mother that they needed to seek help when, after she told him it was bedtime, Luis began crying and rocking himself, saying, "I just wish I were dead."

Two weeks ago, Tanisha woke her parents in the middle of the night, sobbing uncontrollably. She told them that she couldn't stop thinking about killing herself. Tanisha's parents immediately left a message on her outpatient psychiatrist's voice mail and headed to the emergency room. Tanisha was admitted to the child and adolescent psychiatry inpatient unit. She and her family began working with the staff to address her depression.

Talk about suicide is sometimes assumed to be an attempt to get attention. However, recent suicide statistics—such as that the best predictor of a suicide attempt is a history of previous attempts or significant thoughts about suicide—are frighteningly convincing about the need to take suicidal threats seriously.

PUTTING IT ALL TOGETHER

You have just read descriptions of all of the potential symptoms of depression. Some of those descriptions may have sounded a lot like your child. You may want to jot down some notes about which descriptions seemed to fit your child, then continue reading as we go through symptoms of the other mood disorders. As you continue reading this chapter, you'll gain a better sense of where your child fits in. Does your child seem to fit the descriptions of the symptoms of major depression perfectly, or does she experience symptoms of other mood disorders as well? In Chapter 4, we help you understand how the mental health professionals with whom you work will translate the list of symptoms that you and your child describe into a diagnosis.

Dysthymic Disorder

Sixteen-year-old Kendra has been arguing with her mother more and more over the past year. Recently she left the house during an argument and didn't come home for two days. During calm moments her mother has tried asking her what's wrong, but Kendra always says, "Nothing, I'm fine." She spends most of her time sitting around the house. Her mother has encouraged Kendra to get a job or join a school activity, but she just shrugs her shoulders. Kendra spends two hours getting dressed each morning, most of this time is spent trying on outfits, then complaining that she looks awful and that she is ugly. According to her mother, Kendra has seemed somewhat unhappy for as long as she can remember. Kendra's mother is particularly concerned because Kendra's only friend is a girl in the neighborhood who seems to have similar problems. According to Kendra, she likes Jessica because "Jessica understands me."

As with a long-lasting low-grade fever, dysthymic disorder (DD) can be hard to identify because it starts to seem like just a fact of the child's life. A child with DD may have felt mildly depressed for a large percentage of his life and may have begun to identify his typically sad or irritable mood as "normal." Parents and others around the child may have begun to view his irritability or sadness as part of his personality.

Children with DD have a cluster of fewer symptoms than those with MDD, and their mood is usually less severe, but this mood disorder should definitely be treated. Research has indicated that children with dysthymic disorder are ultimately more impaired by their condition than children with MDD, because it's the overall amount of time spent "in episode" (the time during which the child fulfills diagnostic criteria for a disorder) rather than the severity of symptoms that is most clearly associated with long-term outcome. With dysthymic disorder, the symptoms by definition last for at least a year.

Does your child:

■ **Seem sad or unhappy (over a period of at least one year)?**
Neither Kendra nor her mother can remember a time when her mood was brighter. Her mother reported that Kendra "seemed to have a furrowed brow" as an infant.

Kyle is ten. Each day when he wakes up, he says, "This will probably be a bad day." His pessimistic outlook has become so familiar to his parents that they think of it as normal. Kyle just shrugs and says, "I'm not sad, I'm just blah."

■ **Seem irritable (over a period of at least one year)?**
After comparing notes with Jessica's mother, Kendra's mother learned that the two friends have a lot in common regarding mood states and related behavior. Jessica became irritable when she started puberty in fifth grade, and her mother assumed that it was due to "hormones"; but now, five years later, Jessica is still grumbling around the house, snapping at her siblings, and is generally unhelpful and hard to be around. The whole family is tired of her negative mood pervading the house.

▪ Have trouble sleeping?

Kendra has trouble falling asleep, so she stays up late watching TV, then has trouble getting up for school—a constant source of conflict between Kendra and her mother.

Kyle has had trouble falling asleep for so long that he and his parents have developed many coping strategies. He still tosses and turns from 9:00 P.M., when he gets into bed, until 10:00 or 10:30, but at least he no longer comes downstairs four or five times before finally settling down for the night. He has a CD player that can be set to play his favorite CD over and over. His parents turn out his light when they head to bed, as Kyle often falls asleep reading. Finally, they got a kitten so that Kyle would have company in bed.

▪ Seem fatigued?

The school nurse has called Kendra's mother on several occasions because Kendra has fallen asleep during afternoon classes. After school, Kendra often naps some more, which only makes it harder for her to fall asleep at night.

▪ Have a diminished or excessive appetite?

Jessica craves carbohydrates and snacks excessively, especially at night, which has caused her to gain weight. Now she needs new clothes, which Jessica's mother can't afford—another source of conflict between them.

▪ Have low self-esteem or a poor self-image?

Jessica says she isn't good at anything and that she's ugly. She frequently puts herself down and often resists trying new things for fear she won't be able to do them. When her mother enrolled her in an art class at the local community center because Jessica's artwork had won awards at school, which was a great source of pride and enjoyment for her, Jessica's only comment was, "I'm not going. I suck at art."

▪ Have trouble concentrating or thinking?

Even though Kendra was an early reader, writes well (when she gets motivated), doesn't have "math phobia," and did very well through all of elementary school, she has done poorly ever since middle school. Kendra doesn't finish in-class assignments, does poorly on tests, and often doesn't turn in homework assignments.

Kyle has a hard time staying focused on what's going on in class. Although he doesn't disrupt the class, his teachers have noted that he often seems to be in his own world. He does well when his teacher or one of his parents works one-on-one with him, but otherwise he has trouble staying on task. In Kyle's case, it will be important to assess whether his difficulty concentrating is part of his mood disorder or a sign that he also has ADHD. If his concentration difficulties started before his mood problems or if they continue after his mood problems are treated, he may in fact have ADHD, a disorder that commonly co-occurs with mood disorders (see Chapter 4).

■ Express feelings of hopelessness?

When her mother has tried to get Jessica to agree to see a therapist with her, Jessica has resisted because she says that things will never get better anyway.

PUTTING IT ALL TOGETHER

Both MDD and DD can significantly interfere with a child's functioning. If you see a number of the symptoms of depression in your child, you should seek an evaluation even if you aren't sure whether your child fits squarely into one or the other diagnosis. Your child may, in fact, be experiencing both disorders. Children with DD often develop MDD within two to three years and can continue to have dysthymia even when the major depressive episode has resolved. When the dysthymia underlies or continues "below the surface" of major depressive episodes, it is referred to as "double depression."

Bipolar Disorder Type I

Life with thirteen-year-old Mark has always been challenging. He walked and talked very early and never slept much. He was very hard to settle as an infant and toddler, always seemed to sleep less than other children his age, and stopped napping altogether at eighteen months. His mother read every parenting book she could find to help her manage Mark's frequent and extreme tantrums. From preschool through third grade, Mark seemed to enjoy school, although his teachers always described him as "intense" and "high energy." He worked very hard to behave well at school and often had major meltdowns when he got home from school in the afternoon. Fourth grade was a particularly bad year. He went from his usual level of exuberance and even overexcitement to being uninterested in even his favorite activities. For the first time, his teachers started calling home because Mark wasn't completing assignments and was crying frequently in class and on the playground. Mark even started turning down invitations from friends. He was surly around home and weepy at school.

Mark's mother took him to his pediatrician, who started him on an antidepressant and referred him to a child psychologist for therapy. The medication helped, but Mark continued to be frequently irritable and somewhat unpredictable—sometimes being pleasant and positive at home, sometimes being irritable and lashing out for no apparent reason, and sometimes being giggly and overly excited. Over the past year, things have gone from bad to worse. Mark's irritability increased, and he began to have angry outbursts that seemed to come out of the blue and were often directed at family members. His judgment seemed to get worse and worse. One day he went to school with his cousin's parakeet in his jacket; the parakeet escaped and was never seen again. About a month ago, Mark's problems escalated to the point that his parents took him to the emergency room and he was hospitalized. During the week leading up to his hospitalization, Mark's mood ranged from euphoria to angry rage. He called the school superintendent because his teacher and principal did not handle a peer conflict to his satisfaction, and he asked one of the girls in his class if he could touch her breasts in exchange for showing her his penis. He also began talking so fast and changing topics so quickly that his mother couldn't understand him. When she tried to get him to slow down and finish one thought at a time, Mark got furious and threatened her with a kitchen knife. When she and his father tried to drive him to an emergency therapy appointment, Mark attempted to jump out of the car. A call to his therapist confirmed their decision to take him directly to the emergency room.

Bipolar disorder involves cycles between extreme moods at both ends of the spectrum—periods of depression, with extremely low moods (sadness and/or irritability and/or loss of interest), and periods of mania, with extremely high moods (rage or euphoria). Episodes of depression and mania can be separated by years or in some cases by weeks, days, or even hours. (Mark's most significant depressive episode was during fourth grade, at age ten. Now, during seventh grade, at age thirteen, he is having his first full manic episode, although his mood was unstable between ages ten and thirteen.)

Unlike Mark, some kids cycle rapidly between depression and mania, as we described in the section "Understanding Cycling." For others, mania and depression occur simultaneously (a mixed state). During a mixed state, a child might experience anger, agitated excitement, profound sadness, and hopelessness at the same time. This can be extremely difficult for the child, as well as for family members.

The depressive symptoms of bipolar disorder are the same as those for the depressive disorders, described previously. As for mania, some manic symptoms can be very dramatic and frightening. Ask yourself the following questions to recognize mania in your child, keeping in mind that these symptoms vary widely among individuals and age groups.

Does your child:

■ Have periods of elevated or expansive mood?

One week before he was hospitalized, Mark entered his therapist's office shouting, "Today was the best day ever!" When his therapist asked him why, he said, "It just is—I showed them who's boss!" and then giggled uncontrollably for several minutes. Mark proceeded to laugh uproariously as he explained to his therapist that he had been suspended and why.

Behaviors that might indicate an elevated mood include giggling uncontrollably, laughing at inappropriate times, and being "too happy." Prior to his becoming acutely manic, Mark's classmates and family had noticed that he was sometimes strangely exuberant and excited. While working on a group project for his social studies class, Mark was so excited that one of the members of his group asked him to "chill out."

■ Have periods of extreme irritability?

One day Mark came into the kitchen where his mother was preparing dinner. Upon seeing that she was making meat loaf, Mark began screaming and cursing at her. She remained calm and tried to soothe him by offering an alternative meal and talking softly to him. She then tried removing herself from the room. He followed her wherever she went in the house. Despite her efforts, Mark continued to scream and yell for forty-five minutes. Finally he exhausted himself and fell asleep on the couch for an hour.

Prior to the past few weeks, Mark at times would tell his mother that everything was getting on his nerves and that he couldn't stand to be around anyone. On one particular Saturday, he decided to skip his baseball game because he didn't think he could go without getting angry at someone.

During periods of mood change such as those just described, does your child:

■ Express grandiose ideas?

While in the emergency room, Mark explained his plans to earn millions by writing a book that would expose the scandals within his school. He had been keeping notes of his observations of his teachers, classmates, and administrators and thought that he could finish the book by the end of the weekend. Mark thought the book would be a snap to write, and he was sure that his mother would drive him to New York City (a ten-hour drive) so that he could take the book directly to a publisher.

Mark has always had big ideas, but this was the first time one of his ideas has gotten so outlandish and unrealistic. At other times, he has decided to do things that were out of his reach, such as drafting an inaugural address to give when he becomes president and trying to start several businesses.

■ Need less sleep than usual?

At the time of his hospitalization, Mark had slept only eight hours over the previous three days. He told the ER physician that he was not tired and that he was too busy working on his book to take time to sleep. Mark has never seemed to need a lot of sleep (except when he was very depressed during fourth grade and was constantly tired). He has always been the first one up in the house (between 5:00 and 6:00 A.M.) and has gone through periods of not falling asleep until 12:00 or 1:00 A.M. His energy level never seems to be affected by his lack of sleep.

■ Talk more, faster, or louder than usual?

While he was being assessed in the emergency room, Mark's voice got progressively louder, so that he was yelling loud enough to be heard in the waiting area.

Mark's mother noted that it was common for Mark to talk this loudly and quickly, especially when angry or extremely happy and excited. Throughout his time in the emergency room, it was very difficult to interrupt Mark to ask questions or make comments. He spoke so quickly that he had to be stopped periodically and asked to slow down so that he could be understood.

Before things got so much worse, Mark was understandable but always seemed to be on high speed compared with family and friends. He always had lots of ideas and talked fast.

▓ Express or show signs of racing thoughts?

His mother describes Mark as "jumping from topic to topic," during periods of rage. During moments of relative calm, Mark complains about his "brain going too fast."

Some children describe racing thoughts as feeling that their "thoughts are jumping around," that their "thoughts are all jumbled up," or that "someone pushed the fast-forward button on my brain."

▓ Seem more distractible than usual?

During his ER assessment, Mark stopped in the middle of describing the purpose of his planned book to ask about a picture on the wall. He seemed to have difficulty completing a thought without interrupting himself. In addition, his homeroom teacher had called Mark's mother the previous day to express concern that Mark had been turning in incomplete assignments, which was uncharacteristic for him.

It's important to distinguish an increase in distractibility from the distractibility associated with ADHD. Learning has never been a problem for Mark, and he has always been able to focus on school assignments and complete his homework. Becoming distractible is a symptom of mania for Mark. If Mark had a history of ADHD, it would be more difficult to discern whether distractibility was part of his mood disorder or part of his co-occurring ADHD. In such a case, the diagnostician would look for a significant decrease in Mark's ability to concentrate from his usual level of difficulty before counting distractibility as a symptom of mania.

▓ Seem more active or agitated than usual?

Mark's mother described him as being "in perpetual motion." Dinnertime had become a challenge for the family because Mark had begun pacing around the dinner table while everyone was eating, stopping periodically to eat something off his plate.

▓ Act more foolish or reckless than usual?

Mark's decision to take his cousin's parakeet to school is one example of reckless behavior. Another occurred the day before his therapy session, when he approached a girl in his neighborhood and fondled himself while making lewd comments.

In assessing whether a child is exhibiting poor judgment or foolish and reckless behavior, a good rule of thumb is to ask whether the behavior compromised anyone's physical safety—including that of the family pet—or emotional well-being, which includes any behavior that would make others think your child was odd (for example, picking up a microphone during a school assembly and beginning to give a speech without permission).

The course of Mark's bipolar disorder was very typical for bipolar disorder Type I. His problems started out as mild, with sleep difficulties, high energy, and extreme tantrums. He experienced depression before mania, and although his depression lifted once he started taking an antidepressant, his moods continued to be unpredictable, with periods of irritability and periods of elation. When his unstable mood escalated into a manic episode, Mark needed to be hospitalized to keep himself and others safe (he tried to jump out of a moving vehicle and threatened his mother with a knife).

To be diagnosed with BP I, a child must experience a manic or mixed episode that lasts at least one week. In Chapter 4, we provide more details about the diagnostic criteria for BP I.

Bipolar Disorder Type II

Marla is a bubbly eleven-year-old. However, her periods of giggly, silly behavior have begun to get her in trouble at school. Teachers have noticed these episodes and commented to her parents, because Marla is typically a well-behaved and high-achieving student. During these periods Marla talks fast, has many ideas that she feels are brilliant, and starts many projects. Her friends and family find it hard to keep up with her. Marla also goes through times when she is surly and withdrawn at home. Her energy level goes way down, she's difficult to wake for school, and she wants to lie around in bed all weekend. This causes even more problems, because Marla reneges on previous plans she has made, maddening her friends. During these periods she complains that her schoolwork is too hard for her, and it takes her two hours to finish an assignment that would normally take her twenty or thirty minutes. Marla works hard to put on a happy face at school because she doesn't want her friends to see her down, but once she gets home, Marla snaps at family members and has no energy even to play.

Marla was recently diagnosed with bipolar disorder Type II, which involves periods of less severe manic symptoms, called *hypomania*, alternating with depression. Hypomania can be alluring, especially in a child who has been depressed and might just seem to be coming out of the depression. Although hypomania does not lead to the level of problems that typically occur when a child is manic, it represents a change from usual functioning and a mood that is elevated beyond normal levels. A child with hypomania may be able to function in school, with peers, and even at home and may be seen as very funny, dramatic, or energetic—to a degree that makes him or her stand out from the crowd. Although a hypomanic child may be able to function at home, at school, and with peers, she may have significant problems as well. Poor judgment may lead to risky or embarrassing situations. For example, Marla was sure that she deserved the choir solo (despite the fact that the solo is for a soprano and she is an alto). So during choir practice, Marla stepped out in front of the chorus and began singing the solo part at the top of her lungs. The whole chorus stopped singing to watch her while the choir director tried without success to signal her to rejoin the group. Marla also tends to get into awkward situations with peers, such as discussing the invitation list for a party to which she assumed she was invited but was not.

The symptoms of hypomania are identical to those of mania, but the level is less severe and they typically last a shorter period of time (days instead of weeks).

Does your child:

▪ Have periods of elevated or irritable mood that are clearly out of character?

Marla has periods of giddiness and what her mother would describe as "foolish" behavior. During these times, she giggles at everything. Her father finds Marla to be "bubbly" during these times and is not convinced that there is anything wrong with this behavior. At other times, especially if interrupted during one of her projects, Marla can be snippy.

Refer to pages 36–39. Does your child have any of the other behaviors noted under BP I? If your child experiences three or four of the symptoms of mania but for only a few days at a time and if the severity does not seem to match that of full mania, your child may be experiencing hypomania.

Like BP I, BP II is treatable. In Chapter 6 we explore issues related to deciding whether (and when) to try medications. In the case of BP II, this can be a difficult decision, as a child with BP II may do very well at some times and may seem not to need medication, despite problem behaviors at other times.

Cyclothymia

A child with cyclothymia is less likely to come to the attention of professionals because the highs and lows are less severe. In addition, if she does receive an evaluation, the correct diagnosis is easily missed. Cyclothymia is characterized by periods of hypomania and periods of mild depressive symptoms that are not severe enough to be episodes of major depression. These mood changes occur constantly and rapidly with only short and infrequent periods of stable mood (no more than two months).

For as long as twelve-year-old Austin's parents can remember, he has had "sunny days and cloudy days." On his "sunny days" he is happy and sometimes so energetic that his parents and friends have to work to keep up with him. He is enthusiastic about activities and especially interested in new projects. But on his "cloudy days" he is gloomy, slow moving, and hard to get along with. Through elementary school Austin had a close-knit group of friends who knew him well and got used to accommodating his moods. Now that he is in middle school and the social pressure is increasing, Austin is starting to struggle more. Although he still sees his friends from elementary school, they are no longer such a close group. On "up" days, Austin's silly behavior has begun to get him in trouble at school, and on "down" days his peers have no patience with him. Austin's mother received a call from his guidance counselor, who was concerned about his behavior in class. He has been particularly irritable at home—snapping at family members and spending more time than usual in his room.

As we have said previously, your child's mood is a problem when it's a problem. In the case of cyclothymia, mood impairment may not be severe, but it is long lasting and pervades all aspects of life. As a result, it can have devastating effects on development.

Bipolar Disorder NOS (Not Otherwise Specified)

Bipolar disorder NOS is used to describe anyone who experiences significant manic symptoms but who does not fit the descriptions for BP I, BP II, or cyclothymia. As we described previously, there is a significant subset of children with bipolar disorder who experience continuous cycling. These children are often given the diagnosis of BP-NOS.

Eight-year-old Chantelle has constant ups and downs. She has told her mother that she feels "happy-mad-sad," which is her way of describing her constantly changing mood. Chantelle becomes angry with very little warning, then becomes aggressive and destructive. At times her mother has had to hold Chantelle to keep her from hurting herself or someone else. Chantelle can then switch very rapidly to hysterical laughter and hypersexual behavior—masturbating, asking her brother to watch her go to the bathroom, and making comments that would make a sailor blush. Chantelle's mother has racked her brain but cannot think of any time Chantelle could possibly have been sexually abused or been exposed to sexually explicit material. Chantelle's mother has very strict standards about the TV shows watched in their home and monitors Chantelle's friends carefully. In calmer moments, Chantelle's mother has also questioned Chantelle about whether anyone has ever touched her inappropriately, which Chantelle has consistently (and believably) denied. Chantelle also becomes desperately sad and cries over what seems like nothing to those around her. She does dangerous and reckless things, such as running out into the street to race the cars and jumping out of trees convinced that she can land safely no matter how high the jump. So far she has been lucky and hasn't hurt herself seriously.

How Do I Sort Out the Symptoms?

You may have noticed as you read the previous section that some symptoms were listed under more than one diagnostic category. So how do you figure out where your child fits in? Are you dealing with depression or bipolar disorder? Differentiating between the symptoms of mania and depression can often be tricky. In Table 1, we have compared the ways in which symptoms of depression and mania appear.

As we discussed earlier in the chapter, figuring out which mood states your child experiences is the first challenge. Sadness is specific to depression. The one exception is that during a mixed episode (in which depressive and manic symptoms occur simultaneously) sadness can occur along with euphoria.

Irritability can be part of both mania and depression, with the irritability of mania tending to be more intense and episodic. Professionals often struggle with differentiating between the irritability of depression and the irritability of mania. Children with depression may be constantly irritable with no clear "episodes," although they may appear worse dur-

| TABLE 1 | Comparison of Symptoms for Depression and Mania |

Symptoms	Major depression	Mania
Mood state	Sad/irritable/angry	Elevated/expansive/angry
Interest	Loss of interest	Excessive interest in many activities or topics
Sleep	Too much sleep or difficulty sleeping with fatigue	Reduced sleep without fatigue
Appetite	Increased or decreased	—
Thoughts	Morbid or suicidal	Grandiose, rapid
Concentration	Impaired	Impaired
Activity level	Restless or lethargic	Increased
Self-appraisal	Worthless/guilty	Inflated/grandiose
Behavior	Withdrawn/isolated	Reckless or foolish

ing particularly stressful times of day (for example, during the routine of getting ready for school in the morning or when they are hungry or tired). Children with bipolar disorder may also exhibit chronic irritability punctuated by periods of extreme irritability or rage that occur on a daily or weekly basis. These periods of rage may be precipitated by seemingly minor or insignificant events or even seem to come out of the blue (for example, screaming and yelling for forty minutes while throwing things at parents for no apparent reason). During episodes of intense irritability or rage, children can be destructive and verbally and physically aggressive and can have trouble making logical and safe choices. Mania also brings elevated and expansive moods that do not occur during depressive episodes. Your mental health team will help you make the distinction between depression and bipolar disorder by listening to your descriptions and spending time observing and listening to your child.

In some cases, loss of interest can be the primary indicator of depression. Whereas a child with depression would be likely to lose interest in activities, mania tends to bring intensified and often excessive interest in a variety of activities and topics.

Both depression and mania can bring sleep problems. Sleep problems for children with depression can involve a loss of sleep, excessive sleep, or both. When a child with depression has difficulty falling asleep at night, wakes up in the middle of the night, or wakes early in the morning, he typically feels tired, wants to take naps, has trouble getting up, or seems fatigued to others. During mania, the need for sleep often decreases, so that a child sleeps less, often by two or three hours, but does not seem tired and, if anything, is more energetic.

Changes in appetite are not a symptom of mania (although we have seen many children, while manic, make unusual choices of foods to eat). Depression may bring changes in appetite, with either an increase or a decrease, depending on the child.

Content of thoughts can be affected by both depression and mania. Thoughts about death, morbid themes, or suicide can occur during depression. During manic episodes, thoughts are often very rapid and can be grandiose—such as a child believing that she is able to jump from any height and land without getting hurt or believing that she is able to read her teachers' minds.

Changes in ability to concentrate occur in both depression and mania. It may be harder to tell that a depressed child is having difficulty concentrating unless his grades begin to fall, teachers notice a change, or the child complains that he is having trouble focusing. Changes in distractibility may be more evident during mania, based on frequent topic changes and switches between activities.

Changes in activity level frequently occur in depression and mania. Lethargy is specific to depression. However, restlessness or agitation can occur with either mood state. Restlessness or agitation may occur in the form of difficulty sitting still, persistent fidgeting, or pacing. An increase in energy level and episodes of hyperactivity are specific to mania.

Whereas a depressed child would be likely to view herself as worthless or inadequate, a manic child might have an inflated sense of self-worth and may believe himself to be smarter, more attractive, or more talented than is realistic.

A depressed child may be withdrawn and isolate himself. On the other hand, a depressed child who is irritable may have frequent conflicts with peers and siblings and even begin to get into fights at school. Similar behaviors could be seen in a child with bipolar disorder. Reckless or foolish behavior is more typical of mania. The exception may be that a depressed child who is experiencing thoughts about suicide may engage in reckless behavior as a way of hurting herself.

What Is the Mood Disorder and What Are My Child's Traits?

To help your child most effectively, it is important to determine where the mood disorder stops and your child begins. When someone has her first depressive episode at age thirty, her personality, strengths, weaknesses, likes and dislikes, along with her functioning in family and work roles, are well established. They are clearly known to her and to those who care about her. Therefore, if she suddenly goes from being an energetic and happy computer programmer and mother of two to having difficulty getting out bed and crying every night, those around her can see that something is different and wrong. But, if a first depressive episode occurs at age five, ten, or even fifteen, development is still in process. It can become very difficult for family members, friends, and the child himself to figure out who he is and what is or isn't part of him— that is, to distinguish his symptoms from himself. The "enemy" is your child's mood disorder. The mood disorder is what causes your child to struggle at school, at home, and with peers and what generally messes up her life. Once you know your child's enemy, you can begin to fight it.

FAMILY EXERCISE 1: NAMING THE ENEMY

Start with a blank piece of paper and divide it into two columns. Draw or glue your child's picture at the top of the page (an example is provided in Figure 3). Along with your child, begin listing positive items in the left-hand column, including strengths, attributes, and interests. Once this list is complete, begin listing symptoms or problems your child is experiencing or has experienced in the right-hand column. Once both lists are complete, fold the paper in half lengthwise so that the right column covers the left column. This will show both you and your child how mood symptoms cover up all of the good things about your child. Now, unfold the paper and refold it with the symptoms now going behind your child's description. Your child's positive traits are visible again. Just like unfolding the paper, when your child's condition is treated, your child will shine again—and, as you progress in treatment, you and your child will be able to put the problems behind you.

What Is Normal and What Is Not?

DEPRESSED MOOD

Everyone has good days and bad days, so how do you figure out what are ordinary ups and downs and what represent "clinical" ups and downs, or symptoms? For typical children, there should be more good days than bad days, and bad days are likely to have some sort of precipitant or cause.

A Normal Bad Day. Bobby, a seven-year-old, was having a really difficult day. By noon he had started several conflicts with his ten-year-old brother and had already been in tears twice. His mother was at her

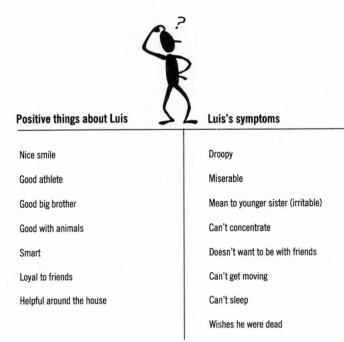

Positive things about Luis	Luis's symptoms
Nice smile	Droopy
Good athlete	Miserable
Good big brother	Mean to younger sister (irritable)
Good with animals	Can't concentrate
Smart	Doesn't want to be with friends
Loyal to friends	Can't get moving
Helpful around the house	Can't sleep
	Wishes he were dead

FIGURE 3 Naming the enemy.

wit's end. Although Bobby and his brother have their fair share of arguments, this was excessive, and Bobby didn't typically behave this way. She was particularly concerned because she has a history of depression and knew that she needed to be on the lookout for symptoms in her boys. When his mother looked at the family calendar later that day, she realized that over the past week they had been out past Bobby's bedtime five days out of seven. He went to bed early that night, and his behavior returned to normal the next day.

A *Pattern of Bad Days.* Recently it seems as though Jenny, a nine-year-old, can barely tolerate having her six-year-old sister in the room without getting angry at her. Getting her to do her homework each night has become a real struggle. Jenny's mother is becoming increasingly frustrated because it feels as though she has more difficult interactions than positive ones with Jenny. To top it off, Jenny's teacher sent a note home requesting a parent–teacher conference because Jenny's grades and behavior are both deteriorating at school.

Shifting Patterns over Time. When your child has a history of a mood disorder, it can be especially difficult to separate normal ups and downs from a recurrence of mood symptoms. Fifteen-year-old Anthony, for example, has experienced severe depression but had been doing well for the past six months. When his mother came home from work one day to find him looking very sad, she immediately got worried and started asking him lots of questions. In response, Anthony became irritable. She decided to wait to see how he was doing the next day before calling his therapist. In the morning Anthony seemed fine, and over breakfast he explained that one of his exams had not gone as well as he had hoped. Anthony asked his mother to please give him a chance to deal with his problems before she panicked and assumed he was relapsing.

However, parents of children with mood disorders do need to be on the lookout for reappearing or worsening symptoms. Dylan is ten and has been doing well on an antidepressant since he became depressed at the age of eight. He did so well in fourth grade that his mother started wondering about discontinuing the medication, but she decided to wait until he was settled in his fifth-grade class. It wasn't until she took Dylan to the pediatrician for a checkup just before Thanksgiving and was questioned by the doctor that she realized that Dylan had become increasingly irritable and down over the past couple of months. Rather than discontinuing his medication, his dose was increased, and he returned to doing well.

MANIC MOOD (EXPANSIVE, ELEVATED, OR IRRITABLE)

How do you tell normal childlike excitement from an elevated or expansive mood? Here are two good questions to ask yourself:

1. Does it fit the situation?
2. Is it causing problems?

A child who is highly excited, giggling, and running around the morning of her birthday party or who wakes the whole house with her excitement on Christmas morning fits the situation (highly exciting events) and probably does not cause any real problems. Compare these scenarios with that of a child who laughs loudly and uncontrollably during a history class, then continues laughing while the principal explains that she is being suspended for disturbing her class. Her elevated mood does not

fit the situation (history class) and is causing problems (she is being suspended from school).

GRANDIOSE BEHAVIOR

It can also be difficult to separate grandiosity from normal child behavior. Again, the same two questions can be used to help make the distinction:

1. Does it fit the situation?
2. Is it causing problems?

For example, make-believe play can sometimes seem grandiose.
Children enjoy pretending to be superheroes and other larger-than-life
characters. This is normal. It occurs during playtime, fits that situation,
and typically does not cause problems. Children also enjoy creating real
and make-believe businesses (for example, a lemonade stand on a hot
day). Creating a lemonade stand, especially with adult assistance, does
not cause any problems; in fact, it can be a positive learning experience.
But a child who takes it upon himself to mow all of the lawns in his sub-
division without asking the various homeowners if they want their lawns
mowed, who mows over flower gardens, and who destroys the lawn
mower in the process is behaving in a way that does not fit the situation
and causes problems. If, instead, this boy had gone door to door on his
street and asked neighbors if they would like their lawns mowed, and if
he had mowed three or four lawns for $10 each, his behavior would be in
the normal realm.

In determining what is normal and what is not, it is better to err on
the side of caution. If you are not sure whether your child's mood and
behavior are consistent with what is termed "within normal limits," seek
consultation. By asking questions of professionals, you are not commit-
ting to anything—you are just getting information that will help you
make good decisions for your child and be your child's best advocate.

DEALING WITH GRIEF

It is normal, in fact expected, for children to react to losses such as divorce, the death of a loved one (including pets), or a close friend moving
away. However, individual children react differently, and it can be diffi-

cult to determine what is a "normal" reaction to a bad event. A child who experiences a loss needs opportunities and help to deal with the loss in a healthy manner. A good rule of thumb is that if your child continues to have difficulty functioning at school, at home, or with peers several months after the event, seek help. Your child may be dealing with very normal feelings, but he is losing out socially and academically.

Whose Disorder Is It?

A tricky complication when determining whether or not your child is experiencing mood symptoms is whether you or your child's other parent has ever experienced mood symptoms. On the one hand, we know that genetics is a major factor in children getting depressed or developing bipolar disorder (this is discussed further in Chapter 3). Besides putting your child at higher risk, this factor means that you (or your spouse or partner) may be exquisitely aware of what it is like to experience these symptoms. Many parents have voiced to us a strong desire that their child not suffer without help as they did when they were children and their symptoms went unrecognized.

On the other hand, parents' desires to spare their children the heartache *they* experienced as children can cause parents to read too much into their children's behavior. Overly scrutinizing your child's every behavior can also produce irritability (as with Anthony, the fifteen-year-old described in the previous section). Rather than playing "20 Questions" with your child on a daily basis, get input from trusted adults—teacher, softball coach, youth minister—who see your child in a setting in which her behavior can be compared with that of her peers.

By now, you may have a clearer sense of the kinds of problems your child is having. After getting a sense of "what," families who consult with us often ask "why" in their next breath. In the next chapter, we share with you what science has taught us about the *whys* of childhood mood disorders. Then, in Chapter 4 we lead you through what you need to do to get your child carefully evaluated.

3 | Why My Child?

Chapter 2 may have cemented your belief that your child is more than just "moody" and may have a mood disorder. Maybe your child's volatility isn't just his "personality," as some well-meaning friends and family have suggested. Perhaps it's not a phase she's going through, as you kept hoping. As a clearer picture of your child's mood patterns emerges, you may start to wrestle with the question of why your child and family are dealing with this problem. What causes mood disorders? Why your child?

If friends, family, and even professionals have suggested that your parenting strategies are at fault, you're not alone. Despite a wealth of research evidence that psychiatric disorders in children, including mood disorders, are not caused by "bad parenting," these myths seem to incubate in hidden corners of our highly scientific world. The truth is that the *cause* of mood disorders is probably in some fundamental way biological. As you'll see in this chapter, however, the *course* of the illness can be greatly influenced by psychosocial events. That is, if your child has a mood disorder, it's not your fault—but it is your challenge.

What we mean is that you can't (well, you *can* but you *shouldn't*) blame yourself for the fact that your child has a mood disorder, but there's a lot you *can* do to influence the quality of your child's treatment plan, his school placement, how well he learns to cope, and how you (and other family members) learn to adjust to his symptoms. We remind you of this point throughout the book. Even though the disorder is not your fault, it *is* up to you to learn how to deal with it. In this chapter we explain what is currently known about the causes of depressive and bipolar disorders, about which elements in a child's life can affect the prognosis, and about what you can do with this information to help your child.

Most parents want to know what causes mood disorders because they're hoping, in their heart of hearts, that if they can pinpoint the cause, they'll be able to find a cure. Identify the type of bacteria causing your child's sore throat and fever, and you can get a prescription for an antibiotic that will wipe it out. Find out your child's headaches are caused by eyestrain and you can get him glasses; discover that they're a consequence of hunger and you can make sure she eats breakfast before school. Unfortunately, it's not that easy with psychological problems. Science has produced a lot more information on the causes and course of psychiatric disorders, especially in adults, in recent years, but there are very few for which we've found a simple cause that can be reversed or eliminated to produce a cure.

Therefore, throughout this book, we focus on *treating the symptoms,* not *curing the illness.* Many different treatments are available for mood disorders, with new, effective interventions emerging all the time. Although we cannot predict who will have another episode and when those episodes will occur, we can teach you how to manage your child's mood disorder.

Lacey had always had some difficulty sleeping and had always been described as "high strung" by those who know her. Third grade turned out to be a particularly difficult year for her. She and her teacher had a personality conflict from the first day of school, and her grandmother became ill in October. By November, Lacey wasn't falling asleep until 12:00 or 1:00 A.M., had begun spending most of her time alone in her room, and seemed unhappy. Her mother recognized the signs of depression in Lacey; she had seen them in her younger sister and her mother while growing up. Although Lacey probably had a biological tendency to become depressed, the stresses in her life brought on, or precipitated, a major depressive episode.

Some stressors may be unavoidable, such as a relative's illness, but some are eminently manageable. Either way, taking steps to reduce stress in a child's life can bring on a corresponding decrease in the frequency and severity of the child's depressive or manic episodes. For example, Lacey's mother might be able to have her switched to a classroom with a teacher who is more compatible with Lacey, and she might get counseling to help Lacey understand and deal with her grandmother's illness. Learning coping strategies to use in response to unavoidable stress can go a long way toward helping a child manage a mood disorder.

Such measures can reduce the likelihood that a child will have another episode or may reduce the intensity or duration of the next episode. We are now acutely aware of the particular importance of preventing the next episode. Recent research has shown that initial episodes are most likely to be brought on by stress but that later episodes are less likely to be triggered by events in a person's life. In addition, later episodes tend to be more severe, and episodes tend to become more frequent.

As you read this book, you will learn ways in which you can influence the course of your child's illness. Effective medications can lessen current symptom severity and prevent or lessen future episodes. Effective therapy can help you and your child develop coping strategies to manage symptoms. You will learn strategies that you and your child can use to help him function at home, at school, and with peers.

A Genetic Link

Mood disorders tend to run in families. The more that scientists learn about genetics, in fact, the more we are coming to understand that psychiatric disorders in general—anxiety disorders, for example—tend to run in families. The same is true for physical health conditions, such as heart disease. And in the same way that family members at risk for heart disease need to be diligent about exercising regularly, eating a low-fat diet, avoiding chronically stressful situations, and not smoking, children who have or are at risk for mood disorders can benefit greatly from managing their own lifestyle choices.

When we ask parents of children with mood disorders about other family members, we often hear about parents, aunts, uncles, and grandparents who either had been diagnosed with mood disorders or who, upon reflection, exhibited some of the symptoms. Take Luis, the seven-year-old with major depressive disorder (MDD) whom you read about in Chapter 2. During his initial evaluation, the psychologist asked Luis's parents whether they had any relatives with mood disorders or symptoms. She drew a family tree that included Luis's grandparents, parents, aunts, uncles, and siblings and asked about each person. When asked in this manner, Luis's parents realized that two of Luis's paternal aunts had experienced significant periods of depression and that his paternal grandfather had often been sullen and angry, suggesting a possible mood disorder. On the maternal side, Luis's grandmother and one of his uncles were described as "excessive worriers," suggesting possible anxiety disorders. Although both of Luis's parents denied any history of their own, his mother later confided privately to the psychologist that Luis's father had struggled with depression through college and that he still had periods during which he was moody and down. Additionally, he used to have a drinking problem that coincided with his difficult college years.

Luis's family illustrates the fact that it may take some careful thought to identify mood disorders in your extended family. We know from scientific studies that if one parent has a mood disorder, the couple's children have a 27 percent chance of developing a mood disorder. That risk increases to 74 percent if both parents have a mood disorder. But how do you determine which behaviors are the consequence of genes and which result from the fact that family members tend to have similar experiences? Researchers have used adopted individuals and twins to figure some of this out.

Adoption Studies

Adoption studies on bipolar disorder show an even stronger genetic determination than exists with other mood disorders. Research has shown that one in three adopted persons *with* bipolar disorder have biological parents with mood disorders. This number compares with one in fifty adopted persons *without* bipolar disorder who have biological parents with mood disorders. These findings suggest that bipolar disorder is passed on through genes rather than through common experiences.

Twin Studies

Another powerful way to determine the effect of genetics on human behavior is through twin studies. Both identical and nonidentical twins share similar experiences and surroundings. However, identical twins have the same genetic makeup, whereas nonidentical twins have no more genes in common than do nontwin siblings. Thus comparing differences between identical and nonidentical twins helps us determine which characteristics are inherited through genes and which are not. Studies have demonstrated that, if one of a pair of identical twins is clinically depressed, a 54 percent chance exists that the other twin will be diagnosed with depression. If one identical twin has bipolar disorder, there is a 67 to 79 percent chance that the other will have bipolar disorder. By way of comparison, if one nonidentical twin has depression, there is only a 19 percent chance that the other nonidentical twin will have depression. Similarly, if one nonidentical twin has bipolar disorder, there is only a 15 to 20 percent chance that other nonidentical twin will as well.

But Why So Young?

Genetics may also help to explain why mood disorders, bipolar disorder in particular, are occurring in younger and younger children. Since 1940, each generation has had a higher rate of mood disorders, and symptoms have appeared earlier than they did in the previous generation. Some research has suggested that an increase in the amount of genetic material that causes a condition (such as bipolar disorder) occurs in each successive generation, which causes symptoms to begin earlier. However, there are many other possible explanations for why mood disorders in children are on the rise in younger and younger children. These include:

- Better detection of mood disorders (although not perfect today, our ability to recognize depression and bipolar disorder in children *far* surpasses our ability to do so a generation ago)
- "Activation" of bipolar disorder by the use of stimulant or antidepressant medication
- Increased stress in family life—divorce rates are sky high, families are highly mobile, and extended-family support is less common than in previous generations
- Possible environmental/toxic exposures that trigger neurochemical reactions in developing brains
- Dietary changes that contribute to increased mood disorders in all ages of individuals

All these explanations are, in part, speculative. Much more research is needed to better understand why we are seeing more and more children with significant mood disorders at a young age.

What Can You Do about It?

You can't choose the genes you get from your parents, and you can't choose the genes you pass on to your children. So, wrangling over whose "fault" it is for passing on "mood genes" is not a very useful way to think about this genetic linkage. But being aware of any family history and sharing that information with clinicians can be helpful.

We know that heart disease is a biological illness that runs in families. We tell our doctors (and our doctors regularly ask) about any family history. Those with a family history are advised to be careful about how they take care of themselves. They might be advised to take an aspirin each day, and they would certainly be encouraged to exercise regularly, eat a healthy diet, and stay away from cigarettes. We use family history of heart disease as an early warning system and as a way to guide treatment. The same goes for mood disorders. You can use your family history to speed up the diagnostic process and to guide treatment.

Understanding What's Happening in Mood Episodes

Once you understand that part of the story is genetics and evaluate your own family history, you may still be left wondering what actually causes mood symptoms to occur. This is a challenging question because the brain is extremely complex and the story underlying mood disorders is still being unraveled. Scientists are increasingly coming to understand that the brains of people with mood disorders differ in significant ways and thus that mood disorders are actual brain disorders.

Carmen was distraught when her fifteen-year-old daughter, Reyna, was hospitalized after she attempted suicide. During a meeting with her daughter's inpatient psychiatrist, Carmen was asked about family history. She confirmed that there was some history of depression in her family. But she still struggled with what was happening to her daughter, who had been so energetic and vibrant until the past few months. The doctor explained that the chemicals, called *neurotransmitters*, that Reyna's brain needed to function properly were not in proper balance. More than likely, her brain did not have enough of the neurotransmitter called *serotonin*. The antidepressant that Reyna had begun taking, Prozac, would increase the amount of serotonin and thus relieve her depression. Although Carmen still had much to adjust to, understanding what was happening and how the medication would help was an important first step.

Whereas deficits in serotonin are involved in depression, excesses of serotonin may be involved in mania. Inadequate amounts of two other neurotransmitters, dopamine and norepinephrine, may also be involved in depression, but excesses of these two chemicals are likely involved in mania. It is important to remember that the brain is complex and that many chemicals interact in numerous parts of the brain to cause depression and mania. Many studies have shown that some areas of the brain are less active during depression—especially the front part of the brain, which is involved in regulating activity—and that the parts of the brain that regulate emotion are different in individuals with mood disorders.

Using What You Know

Family history can help your treatment providers in the diagnostic process and can sometimes help to guide medication choices. For example, knowing that a child who is experiencing only symptoms of depression has a family history of bipolar disorder raises the clinician's awareness that what currently looks like depression might turn out to be bipolar disorder. In a case like this, the prescribing physician might choose medications carefully to avoid causing manic symptoms (some antidepressants are more likely to set off manic symptoms, whereas stimulant medications can cause agitation or trigger psychosis in a person with bipolar disorder). If a close relative has had symptoms similar to your child's and has done particularly well with a certain medication, that medication might be a good first choice for your child.

WHO IS AT RISK FOR BIPOLAR DISORDER?

If your child is depressed, you may be wondering whether she is at risk for developing bipolar disorder. Boris Birmaher and his colleagues at Western Psychiatric Institute in Pittsburgh have reported that about one-fourth to one-half of depressed children develop bipolar disorder within two to five years of their developing depression. Certain factors suggest a greater risk for developing bipolar disorder—lethargy (i.e., feeling slowed down), sleeping too much, and experiencing psychotic symptoms while depressed. Having a family history of bipolar disorder or a history of multiple family members with any mood disorder also increases the risk. Becoming hypomanic after starting antidepressant medication creates an additional risk factor for developing bipolar disorder.

Moving On

In some cases, learning about family history helps to answer your own nagging questions of "Why me?" or "Why my child?" Once you've dealt with those questions, you can move on to doing everything in your power to control the course of your child's illness.

Jeremiah had been having periods of very agitated behavior alternating with periods of extreme sadness. As his behaviors became more and more extreme, his mother, Cassandra, spoke to his pediatrician. In addition to suggesting that Jeremiah be evaluated by a child and adolescent psychiatrist, the pediatrician asked if there was any family history of bipolar disorder. Cassandra's initial answer was no. During the two months until Jeremiah could be seen by the specialist, she thought a lot about the pediatrician's question. Her grandfather had been a heavy drinker, and she had always assumed that his periods of anger were related to alcohol. Could they have been related to bipolar disorder? One of her brothers never seemed to be able to keep a job and had always been moody. What about him? No one in her family had ever been diagnosed (to her knowledge) with a mood disorder, but maybe there was more family history than she had thought. By the time of Jeremiah's appointment, Cassandra had made some careful notes that included answers to questions she had begun to ask of her extended family, as well as her in-laws. In so doing, Cassandra learned that her brother had been seeing both a therapist and a psychiatrist and that he had begun taking a

---

FAMILY EXERCISE 2: DRAWING YOUR FAMILY TREE

Figure 4 shows how a family history can be generated using a family tree. You may want to go through this exercise to get a better sense of what, if any, mood disorders run in your family. Include all the biological relatives of your child on both sides of the family when you construct your family tree. This is important, even if your child does not know or has not had recent contact with some of his relatives. If your child is adopted, record whatever birth family history you have available to you. In addition to asking about mood disorders, you might want to note whether any family members have had problems with anxiety, hyperactivity, impulsivity, alcohol or drug abuse, or other emotional or behavioral concerns. Start at the bottom left side of the page and draw in your children (oldest to youngest). Use squares for males and circles for females. Next, draw in yourself and your children's other parent above the children (usually when drawing these, we put fathers on the left and mothers on the right). Add your siblings and the siblings of your children's other parent (your children's aunts and uncles). Finally, add your children's grandparents (your parents and the parents of your child's other parent). Once everyone is drawn in, think about all these people. Is there anyone who has any of the symptoms described in Chapter 2? Is there anyone you think of as having "problems"? If you don't know diagnoses, just write down brief descriptions of each person in your family tree (e.g., "At times, Anna stayed in her room alone for long periods"). Use Figure 4 as a guide.

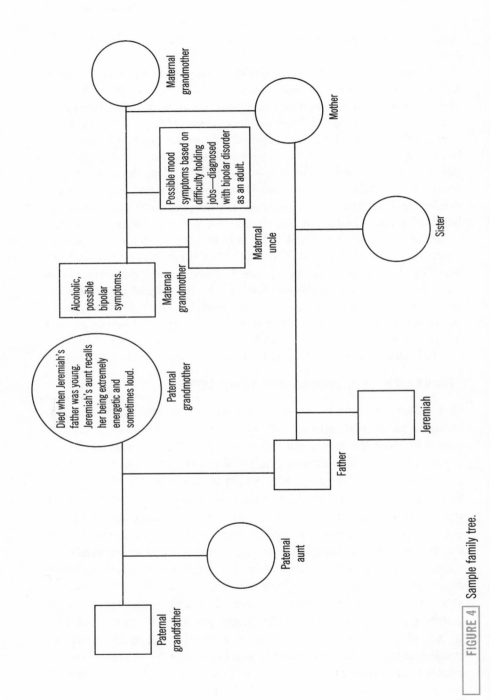

Paternal grandfather

Paternal aunt

Paternal grandmother

Died when Jeremiah's father was young. Jeremiah's aunt recalls her being extremely energetic and sometimes loud.

Father

Jeremiah

Alcoholic, possible bipolar symptoms.

Maternal grandmother

Maternal uncle

Possible mood symptoms based on difficulty holding jobs—diagnosed with bipolar disorder as an adult.

Maternal grandmother

Mother

Sister

FIGURE 4   Sample family tree.

mood stabilizer about two years ago. He had been doing much better over the past eighteen months. When the psychiatrist asked about family history, Cassandra was able to provide very useful information, most of which she had not known when her pediatrician had asked her similar questions two months earlier.

Although we know that genes play a role in determining who develops mood disorders, they don't play the entire role. Nearly half of the story isn't fully known. You probably can't change what causes your child's mood disorder, but you *can* make a difference in its course. You can start with acceptance—accepting that your child's underlying biology (along with yours and those of your family members) cannot be changed.

Marsha knew something was wrong from the time Bobby was about three. Her two older children had certainly had tantrums, but Bobby's were so much more severe and seemed to happen much more often. Finally, after a particularly bad week, she made an appointment with Bobby's pediatrician, who referred her to a psychologist. Marsha went to the first appointment without Bobby. She cried through most of the hour as she described Bobby's problems, her own history of depression, and her ex-husband's history of extreme mood swings—all things that had kept her up late worrying and unable to sleep. Marsha left the appointment feeling relieved to have shared her fears. On the drive home she resolved to take action: She would learn all she could about Bobby's problems and help him however she could.

Once you've stopped the "blame game," you can move forward far more productively to seek solutions to your child's problems. In subsequent chapters we give you suggestions to optimize your child's evaluation and her subsequent treatment and to guide you through ways to get the best possible evaluation and to prepare for the evaluation and for subsequent appointments. Additionally, we give you suggestions about making a number of environmental adjustments (for example, reducing family conflict by improving communication and problem solving, especially in regard to managing your child's symptoms) to change the course of your child's illness.

Accepting your child's biology and recognizing that blaming yourself or anyone else is harmful are the beginning of what we call *deguiltifying*. Again, we go back to our motto: It's not your fault, but it is your challenge. So resolve to take action: You can make a difference, and your first challenge is to get a thorough evaluation.

4 The First Step in Getting Good Treatment Is Getting a Good Evaluation

Up to this point you've learned a lot about what childhood mood disorders look like and why they occur. You may be formulating a good sense of where your child fits into the diagnostic picture. Now you need to know how to start getting help for your child. Your first step is to have your child thoroughly evaluated by a competent mental health professional. This chapter provides you with the information you need to navigate each step of the evaluation process.

Diagnoses of mood disorders in children can be difficult to establish and need to be made carefully. As you work with a mental health practitioner in identifying what's wrong with your child, keep the following points in mind, making sure that they have all been taken into account in arriving at conclusions:

1. *Children are constantly changing—physically, cognitively, and emotionally.* Is the four-year-old who has begun to throw more frequent and intense tantrums expressing irritability as a symptom of a mood disorder or starting to assert his independence and test limits? Diagnosing a moving target is harder than diagnosing one that is standing still. Make sure that an evaluation of your child looks at apparent mood-related behavior in the context of the child's behavior over his or her entire history.

2. *Although children can be quite good at showing us how they feel, they are unlikely to express it verbally in direct terms.* Rather than

saying "Hey, Mom, I'm really depressed," they are likely to say "I hate school!" or "I'm bored!" Many kids don't use words at all—their behavior says it for them. They might start getting into more trouble at school or they might become uninterested in their friends and activities. When they do speak, they tend to use concrete or literal descriptions—phrases such as "My brain feels like it is stuck in the mud" or "My ideas are having a race" might describe slowed thinking or racing thoughts, respectively. An added challenge is that often children either do not understand that things could be different or have never known anything different, so that if you ask them "What's wrong?" they'll say "Nothing." An astute clinician—like a sensitive parent—will know how to interpret your child's statements based on his or her overall behavior and emotional state.

3. *The symptoms of mood disorders are sometimes exaggerations of normal child behavior (at some developmental stages) or behavior that is normal in some situations.* Typical eight-year-olds climb trees while pretending to be Spiderman. In contrast, a child who announces to his fourth-grade class that he has superpowers and then proceeds to climb on a desk and trries to swing from the light fixture is more likely manic. Similarly, temper tantrums are a normal part of a child's testing of her environment during the preschool years. Temper tantrums become symptoms when they reach excessive levels, continue to occur frequently, and increase rather than decrease in intensity and duration by school age. The professional who evaluates your child must take the child's age and developmental stage into account and must be able to view the child's behavior along a continuum of frequency, severity, and duration to determine whether it is cause for concern.

Finding the Right Clinician

How do you find a clinician who can meet the challenges we just described? Consider the following criteria.

Is the Practitioner Qualified?

There are two things you need to know before scheduling an evaluation with a clinician: Is the individual familiar with depression and bipolar disorder? Does she have experience working with children in your child's age range who have mood disorders? Working with elementary school-age children is different from working with adolescents; likewise, working with school-age children is different from working with pre-schoolers.

Is the Fit Good?

Just as important as finding a qualified practitioner is finding one with whom you can develop a trusting relationship. Do you feel comfortable talking with this clinician? This person may become your lifeline during moments of crisis, and you may need to seek advice about sensitive topics. If you're not comfortable and hold back information or concerns, you won't get the best possible service. Although some of your child's behavior may be embarrassing to you, your clinician needs to know these "family secrets" to best provide help to your child and your family.

Cassandra was hesitant to report some of six-year-old Jeremiah's behavior (explicit sexual comments toward his mother, rubbing up against the family dog, exposing himself to his sister) because she was afraid either that sexual abuse would be suspected or that her parenting would be questioned. Compounding the issue were horror stories she had heard about the children's services agency taking children away from their parents. As she became more comfortable during the evaluation, Cassandra described Jeremiah's behavior. She was relieved when the clinician reassured her and explained that those behaviors were symptoms of mania.

Will It Be Practical to See This Practitioner?

- Do the individual's hours fit your schedule? Or can you change your schedule to be able to attend sessions?
- Is the person on your provider list and covered by insurance? Or can you negotiate with your insurance to make an exception to its provider panel, if no one else on its local list has expertise in treating childhood mood disorders?
- Can you afford the cost of sessions? Even with insurance coverage, you may be responsible for a percentage of the cost.
- Can you get to the clinician's office on a regular basis? The best clinician in the world won't do you any good if you can't see him as often as necessary.

If it is inconvenient to see the expert clinician you have found weekly or biweekly, consider continuing with that person through the evaluation process. A thorough evaluation is necessary before a good treatment plan can be developed, and dealing with a long drive, difficult scheduling, or some out-of-pocket expenses might be worth the trouble if it means getting your child the highest quality comprehensive evaluation available in your area. Then you and the evaluating clinician can develop an intervention plan that includes providers more convenient or more affordable for you.

Who Are the Players in the System?

When you're about to choose a clinician to evaluate your child, it's a good idea to understand which mental health professionals are trained to do what. Job functioning may differ somewhat from locale to locale, and practice styles will differ from one clinician to another, but the descriptions that follow represent ways in which many practitioners conduct evaluations and/or provide treatment.

Psychiatrists

A psychiatrist is a medical doctor (MD or DO) with special training in psychiatry. Child and adolescent psychiatrists have completed standard adult psychiatry training and have received further training with children and teenagers. Although psychiatrists have had some training in conducting therapy, their main roles usually are to complete diagnostic evaluations, make medication recommendations, and follow up with pharmacological treatment. An evaluation done by a psychiatrist is likely to involve interviews with parent(s) and the child and possibly the completion of rating scales by parent(s) and/or teachers. Sometimes medical tests, such as a check of thyroid levels or a computerized tomography (CT) scan of the head, will be ordered. If the psychiatrist recommends treatment with medication, he or she will ask you to schedule follow-up appointments. The frequency of follow-up appointments will depend on how your child is doing (for example, is your child in crisis and having trouble functioning from day to day, or is your child managing adequately at school with tolerable functioning at home?). Until your child is stable, appointments may be scheduled anywhere from one to four weeks apart. Once your child is stable, the frequency may be reduced to once every one to three months. Sometimes appointments are scheduled once every six months if symptoms have been managed successfully and an existing medication regimen is just being maintained. Many psychiatrists consult with primary care physicians, such as pediatricians, to provide routine follow-up care after the initial diagnosis is made and treatment regimen begun. In these cases, it is useful for the psychiatrist to monitor progress every six or twelve months or so in case dosage adjustments are needed.

Psychologists

A psychologist has earned a doctorate in psychology (PhD or PsyD) and can also conduct an evaluation. As with the psychiatrist, the evaluation will involve interviews with both you and your child and may include the completion of rating scales. Depending on the questions or concerns that you raise, a psychologist may do cognitive testing, or psychoeducational testing, usually when a child is having difficulty at school. However, this testing is more accurate once a child's mood symptoms have gotten somewhat better, because depression, behavioral problems, and mania can interfere with your child's test performance.

Neuropsychologists are psychologists who specialize in detailed testing of specific cognitive abilities. A neuropsychological evaluation will provide assessments of specific areas—such as visual, verbal, and problem-solving abilities—and an analysis of strengths and weaknesses. Although many children with mood disorders do not require this specialized testing, it can sometimes lead to useful recommendations, particularly if your child has also experienced head trauma or an illness that can affect brain functioning.

In addition to the evaluation, a psychologist can provide individual therapy, family therapy, and parent guidance. For children and adolescents with mood disorders who are being treated with medication, collaboration with the prescribing physician is also important. Contact between providers may be only periodic, but because the psychologist usually will have more time with you and your child than the prescribing physician will, she can sometimes provide important information to that treatment team member, especially if the physician is your pediatrician or family doctor.

A psychologist may also communicate with the educational team. This may take the form of writing letters, providing written reports, or having periodic phone conversations with teachers, guidance counselors, or administrators. Your psychologist is unlikely to be able to attend school meetings due to scheduling constraints. Additionally, few if any insurance companies reimburse professionals for time at school meetings. Sometimes special arrangements can be made, especially if you are able to pay for the psychologist's time and transportation or if school personnel are able to come to your psychologist's office with you. If your psychologist has not been involved with educational issues and you feel that you need help, ask.

Social Workers

A social worker typically has a master's degree, occasionally a PhD, in social work. She will also have a variety of letters after her name, such as LISW (licensed independent social worker). Social workers may conduct diagnostic evaluations. In many clinics, social workers serve as *gatekeepers* for psychiatric services. This means that you would be scheduled for an evaluation with a social worker prior to seeing a psychiatrist. Social workers also provide individual therapy, family therapy, or parent guidance and also should collaborate with the prescribing physician. A social worker may also communicate with the educational team. Again, if you need help in establishing your child's educational services, ask for it.

Counselors

Depending on the state in which you live, you may encounter a variety of different mental health professionals who are likely to be referred to as counselors (e.g., licensed professional clinical counselor, or LPCC). These individuals will vary in their training and experience but are likely to have the equivalent of a master's degree. Like social workers, they may serve as gatekeepers for psychiatric services and are also likely to provide therapy. As with the other providers we've discussed, their helpfulness will depend on their experience with mood-disordered children in your child's age range.

Case Managers

The role of the case manager is to help coordinate services. A case manager is not typically provided unless your child has had very serious problems and has not been able to function at home or at school. Multiple hospitalizations often result in the assignment of a case manager. Case managers typically work through a mental health center or family services agency through which your child may be receiving other care. Unlike psychiatrists, psychologists, and social workers, case managers will work with your child individually at your child's school or at your home. A case manager is also likely to work with parents on strategies for managing problems at home and may work with the educational team to coordinate services. A case manager is more likely to be available to attend educational meetings. The training and skills of case managers will vary significantly. They may not have specific expertise in mood disorders.

Home-Based Therapists

The role of the home-based therapist is to work with your child and family within the home to improve communication and behavior and to manage crises. To get a home-based therapist, you usually need to be working with an agency that provides this service. There is considerable variability among communities regarding the availability of home-based therapists. The degrees and training of home-based therapists can differ widely.

Inpatient Hospital Teams

Children and adolescents with mood disorders sometimes require hospitalization. The hospital provides a safe place during times of severe symptoms that make the child a danger to himself or others. Hospitalization is sometimes also used when the evaluator wishes to conduct many medical tests or to determine how the child might function in a different environment. The inpatient team is made up of doctors, nurses, social workers, educational staff, and psychiatric aides. The goal of inpatient hospitalization is to achieve stabilization and then discharge for follow-up (usually within a week) to outpatient therapy and medication management (by your psychiatrist and psychologist). Medications are likely to be adjusted during a hospital stay, and a limited number of family therapy sessions may also occur.

Day Treatment or Partial Hospitalization

These programs are also typically short (one to two weeks). In them children arrive at and depart from the hospital setting during a work day. Services provided during partial hospitalization are similar to inpatient hospitalization services.

Regardless of who conducts your initial evaluation (social worker, psychologist, psychiatrist), you may ultimately need to have a team of mental health providers. In Part II of this book we discuss treatment in detail. For now, we want to make sure you understand who will be conducting your child's evaluation and how to prepare for it. Part of being a good consumer is seeking clarification. If you are unsure what role a particular provider will play in your child's care, don't hesitate to ask.

Preparing for the Evaluation

Finding the best possible clinician is a great first step, but you can also do a little homework to ensure the most productive evaluation possible. Here are some ideas about what information you should organize prior to the first appointment.

- When did problems start? When did you first notice symptoms? When did particular symptoms start?
- What stressful life events has your child experienced? Make sure you include losses such as deaths of significant people or pets, moves, school changes, or illnesses of family members. Keep in mind that any significant change is stressful even if the event isn't "bad" (e.g., starting school; moving, even within the same school district; remarriage of a parent; birth of a sibling). You may find it helpful to make a timeline—Figure 5 shows Jeremiah's as an example.

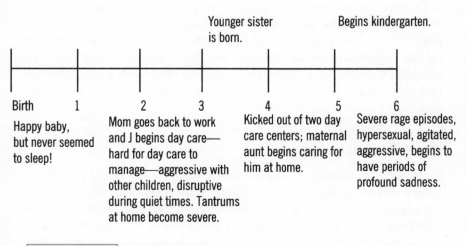

FIGURE 5 Jeremiah's timeline.

- How has your child developed? When did he or she walk and talk? How has your child's social development unfolded compared with peers (e.g., does your child play well with other children his or her age)?
- Does your child have any notable medical history? Unusual or serious illnesses? Chronic conditions? Injuries? Hospitalizations?
- How has school gone for your child? Before your child's evaluation is a good time to talk with teachers to get a sense of how he is doing academically, behaviorally, and socially. Find out how he behaves during structured and unstructured times (e.g., on the playground).
- Does your child have any family members with diagnosed or undiagnosed mental illnesses? In Chapter 3 we discussed the importance of family histories in more detail.
- Has your child had any previous testing, evaluations, or mental health treatment? Be sure to bring copies of any prior evaluation or testing reports. It can be helpful for a new provider to know what you've tried previously, including what interventions have and have not worked (e.g., therapy; specific medications, including dosages, your child has taken).

Know yourself—do you need to write information down in order to be organized? The clinician conducting the evaluation is likely to ask many questions similar to those described here. These questions may help you say everything that you want to say, but they also may not. If there are details you think are particularly relevant, make a list for yourself so that you remember to share them with the clinician.

Some clinicians will mail out questionnaires for you to complete prior to your first visit. These can be very helpful, because they will give you an opportunity to think about questions that might not have occurred to you otherwise. Whether or not your clinician follows that practice, you should take some time to prepare before your first appointment.

Mood Records

Especially if your child's mood changes frequently, you might find that it is very difficult to describe the volatility you experience without sounding vague ("He's always 'flipping' his emotions") or exaggerating ("There is never a calm moment with Dominique!"). Keeping a daily log of your child's moods can make the initial evaluation and future mental health visits more efficient by helping you convey an accurate description of mood fluctuations, as well as the severity of your child's moods.

Jeremiah was referred for a psychiatric evaluation by his pediatrician after his mother, Cassandra, described his increasingly volatile mood and aggressive behavior toward her. In preparation for the evaluation, Cassandra began tracking his mood twice a day, using 10 to describe his worst moods, 5 to indicate a tolerable but unpleasant mood, and 1 to describe moments of normal mood. Cassandra maintained mood records for the two weeks prior to his appointment. For the most part, Jeremiah had 8's, 9's, and 10's, with mornings and afternoons/evenings characterized primarily by angry moods or rages, accompanied by some sadness and some euphoria. It was challenging for Cassandra to complete her ratings each day, but the daily ratings provided a clear picture of Jeremiah's moods and how serious the situation had become. Based on Cassandra's descriptions, observations of Jeremiah in the office, and the mood ratings she'd provided, the psychiatrist made a diagnosis of bipolar disorder and started Jeremiah on a mood stabilizer. Cassandra left the visit feeling that she had made an important contribution to the diagnostic process.

Mood records can also help you track your child's progress once treatment has begun. Once Jeremiah had started on Depakote, Cassandra continued tracking his mood twice daily for the two weeks leading up to his second visit with the psychiatrist. The day before the appointment, Cassandra felt frustrated and hopeless and was ready to tell the psychiatrist that the medication wasn't working, until she sat down to review the mood chart. Then she realized that although he still had 8's, 9's, and 10's, her son had started to have some 4's, 5's, and 6's, too. Obviously they still had a way to go, but she recalled that the psychiatrist had warned her that some dosage increases would probably be needed to get the greatest effect. Cassandra realized that living with Jeremiah day to day had made it difficult to reflect on his overall pattern of improvement, as she still was in the midst of a very rough time with her son.

Sometimes improvements are difficult to see, especially if your child continues to have severe moods. Initial improvements may take the form of slightly less severe mood swings or less frequent or less intense rages. Pay attention to the *frequency* of the mood swings (how often they occur), as well as their *duration* (how long they last) and *severity* (how intense they are).

Keeping careful records helps you notice whether or not your child's condition is getting better, but admittedly it can feel like a lot of work—especially because it's probably most important to keep them during times when you're most stressed by your child's symptoms. At the very least, try to keep mood records before your child's evaluation, because they can be very helpful in graphically representing your child's mood cycles and the relative severity of the symptoms from day to day—important factors in making a diagnosis.

We've included three examples of charts for recording your child's mood. You can photocopy whichever version fits your needs.

The most basic mood record (Figure 6) has spaces for you to make one daily rating indicating whether your child is doing well (10), so-so (5), or terrible (0). Note the day of the week (M, T, W, Th, F, S, Su) to help sort out patterns. For some children, mood improves during the week, when they have the structure of school. For others, mood improves over the weekend, when the stress of school is removed. Also keep track of any important changes or events. You can also use this form as a maintenance chart to help you catch new episodes early.

The second mood log (Figure 7) provides spaces for you to track sad, angry, and happy/euphoric moods once per day. This level of complexity is necessary only if your child experiences different mood states.

The third log (Figure 8) provides spaces for you to track sad, angry, and happy/euphoric moods twice per day. This is the most complex record and is necessary only for children who seem to have significant differences between their morning and afternoon/evening moods.

Write Down Your Questions and the Answers

We've probably all had the experience of leaving our doctor's office only to realize we never asked the question that's been nagging at us for the past couple of weeks. The best antidote is to start writing down your questions before appointments. Some parents are afraid they'll appear stupid if they have to read from a "cheat sheet," but it's too easy to forget your important questions when you're in the doctor's office trying to absorb all the information and advice being offered. Virtually no one remembers everything they wanted to ask without this aid. The same goes for the answers: What your clinician says in the office may make perfect sense at the time, but you may not remember the details of her comments if you don't write them down. Doing so will give you a chance to review the information and think about it later.

The best system of all, we've found, is to have one notebook or binder that you take to all your appointments. Keep a separate section for each provider (e.g., psychiatrist, social worker, psychologist). This is also a good place to keep copies of reports and any other papers about your child and his or her treatment. This will assist you in remembering

Child's name: _____ Month: _____ Treatment providers/programs: _____

Medications (type, dose, side effects): _____

Day	Date	Overall rating*	Comments (e.g., life event, med. changes med. side effects, sleep/appetite changes, other)
	1		
	2		
	3		
	4		
	5		
	6		
	7		
	8		
	9		
	10		
	11		
	12		
	13		
	14		
	15		
	16		
	17		
	18		
	19		
	20		
	21		
	22		
	23		
	24		
	25		
	26		
	27		
	28		
	29		
	30		
	31		

*1 = terrible; 5 = so-so; 10 = great

FIGURE 6. Basic Mood Record.

Child's name: _____

Month: _____ Treatment providers/programs: _____

Medications (type, dose, side effects): _____

Day	Date	Sad	Angry	Euphoric	Meds. taken?	Comments (e.g., life event, med. changes, side effects, sleep/appetite changes, other)
	1					
	2					
	3					
	4					
	5					
	6					
	7					
	8					
	9					
	10					
	11					
	12					
	13					
	14					
	15					
	16					
	17					
	18					
	19					
	20					
	21					
	22					
	23					
	24					
	25					
	26					
	27					
	28					
	29					
	30					
	31					

Rate each mood state for appropriate time periods, with 1 = normal/healthy and 10 = worst/inappropriate to situation.

FIGURE 7 Mood Record: Tracking three moods, once a day.

Child's name: ______________________

Month: __________ Treatment providers/programs: ______________________

Medications (type, dose, side effects): ______________________

Day	Date	Sad A.M.	Sad P.M.	Angry A.M.	Angry P.M.	Euphoric A.M.	Euphoric P.M.	Meds. taken?	Comments (e.g., life event, med. changes, med. side effects, sleep/appetite changes, other)
	1								
	2								
	3								
	4								
	5								
	6								
	7								
	8								
	9								
	10								
	11								
	12								
	13								
	14								
	15								
	16								
	17								
	18								
	19								
	20								
	21								
	22								
	23								
	24								
	25								
	26								
	27								
	28								
	29								
	30								
	31								

Rate each mood state for appropriate time periods, with 1 = normal/healthy and 10 = worst/inappropriate to situation.

FIGURE 8 Mood Record: Tracking three moods, twice a day.

when your last appointment was and provide you with one common place to write down questions before your next appointment, to briefly jot down lab values or test results, and to record answers to questions while you're at your appointments. If your spouse or your child's other caregiver(s) cannot attend the session, this provides a good way for you to update them on your child's progress in treatment. Your provider will also appreciate that you're organized and actively engaged in the treatment process.

Making the Diagnosis

With the information provided by you, your child's other parent, your child, observations made during the evaluation, and any information provided by other sources such as your child's teacher, the evaluating clinician will use established diagnostic criteria to determine the appropriate diagnosis or diagnoses for your child. In some cases you will leave the evaluation with a clear diagnosis. Often, however, the initial appointment is only the beginning of an evaluative process. You may hear the term *working diagnosis,* which means that, although your child's exact diagnosis needs to be confirmed, this is the diagnosis (or diagnoses) that most accurately describes your child. For example, your clinician may tell you that because you reported several symptoms of mania and depression, your child's working diagnosis is bipolar disorder but that more observation over time is needed to be sure. You may also hear the term *rule-out diagnosis.* This means that there is significant reason to consider the diagnosis but that your clinician wants to watch for additional signs and symptoms to develop over time before making a firm diagnosis. Your child might be given a rule-out diagnosis of major depressive disorder (MDD) if, for example, the child meets the diagnostic criteria for depression but your clinician, having noted some possible physical problems, wants to do some lab tests before making a definitive diagnosis of MDD.

In the United States, diagnostic criteria come mainly from the American Psychiatric Association's *Diagnostic and Statistical Manual* (fourth edition; DSM-IV). This manual is updated periodically based on observations made by clinicians and researchers that have helped establish specific rules for the diagnosis of each mood disorder. The criteria establish which specific symptoms must be present and how many symptoms overall must be present to make a particular diagnosis. In addition, the minimum duration for each disorder is specified. As the mental health field gains knowledge about various psychiatric disorders, the criteria evolve. It is the evaluating clinician's job to stay up to date on such changes. Becoming generally familiar with the criteria for each diagnosis will better equip you to provide information during the evaluation and will give you a sense of whether the diagnosis the clinician makes seems accurate. The right diagnosis is important because the diagnosis will steer treatment decisions. Also, diagnoses provide a common language for talking about a particular condition.

As you read the following descriptions, see if the pattern you observe in your child seems to fit any of the diagnoses listed. Jot down questions you will want to ask if the doctor diagnoses your child with any of these disorders.

Major Depressive Disorder

The symptoms of MDD appear in the accompanying sidebar. To be diagnosed with MDD, a child must have had these symptoms for at least two weeks, but in reality few children come to clinical attention after only two weeks of symptoms. It's difficult for most parents to notice a pattern of symptoms clustering together after such a short time, and even once they do, it can easily take several weeks to get an appointment with a clinician. Typically, a lot more time elapses before a child is diagnosed with major depression. The average length of an episode of depression in a child is seven to nine months—the equivalent of most or all of a school year in the life of a child. By one-and-a-half to two years, 90 percent of depressed children have gotten well, but 6 to 10 percent continue to have symptoms and difficulty functioning. Of those who get well, 40 percent have another episode within two years, and 70 percent have another episode within five years.

MAJOR DEPRESSIVE DISORDER

Symptoms must occur for at least two weeks.

A. Either or both:
 1. impaired mood (sad or irritable)
 2. loss of interest

B. Three to four of the following symptoms:
 1. increased or decreased appetite
 2. increase or decrease in sleep (with fatigue)
 3. restlessness or lethargy
 4. fatigue or loss of energy
 5. feelings of worthlessness or excessive guilt
 6. loss of concentration or inability to make decisions
 7. thoughts about death or suicide

These statistics are important—they remind us about the importance of treatment and of paying attention to how your child is doing so that you catch recurrences early.

Dysthymic Disorder

As described in Chapter 2, dysthymic disorder (DD) is what we call the "low-grade fever" of mood disorders. To meet criteria for DD, your child's symptoms must have lasted for one year or longer.

DYSTHYMIC DISORDER

For children, symptoms must last for at least one year (two years for adults).

A. Impaired mood (sad or irritable) for at least one year

B. Two or more of:
  1. poor appetite or eating too much
  2. insomnia or sleeping too much
  3. fatigue or low energy
  4. low self-esteem
  5. poor concentration or trouble making decisions
  6. hopeless feelings

Dysthymic disorder can begin to feel like a fact of life. A child whose mood has been dysphoric for as long as he can remember might not be able to describe his mood or might say that nothing is wrong simply because he does not remember ever feeling any different. If DD is not treated, a single episode will last four years on average. A major depressive episode usually comes two to three years after DD starts, and 13 percent of children with DD develop bipolar disorder. In addition, 15 percent of children and adolescents with DD develop substance abuse problems.

Depressive Disorder Not Otherwise Specified

Whenever an individual has some significant features of a disorder but doesn't fit the criteria, the term *NOS*, meaning "not otherwise specified," is used. *Depressive disorder NOS* can be used to describe a child who has some significant depressive symptoms but who doesn't match the criteria for major depression or dysthymic disorder. As one example, depressive disorder NOS may be diagnosed when significant depressive symptoms occur but the length of the episode does not meet criteria for MDD or DD.

Alicia is twelve years old. Ever since starting middle school seven months ago, Alicia has had periods of being very sad, during which she also has trouble sleeping, loses her appetite, talks about wanting to die, and cannot concentrate on her schoolwork—five of the symptoms required for a major depressive episode—but the episodes last only two or three days. Given that Alicia is twelve and may have begun menstruation, the timing of these two- to three-day periods should be considered carefully. If her symptoms occur primarily in the week prior to menstruation, she may meet criteria for premenstrual dysphoric disorder.

Similarly, depressive disorder NOS would be diagnosed if the symptoms are of adequate severity and duration but are not numerous enough for a diagnosis of major depression.

Marcus is a fifteen-year-old high school sophomore who was doing fine until November. Throughout November, however, he became increasingly sad and had more and more trouble falling asleep each night, eventually finding himself lying awake until 1:00 or 2:00 A.M. Fatigue made school and the cross-country team more and more difficult, and his grades slipped from A's to B's. Marcus's primary care physician checked him carefully for anemia and other health concerns, but his low energy and fatigue appeared to flow from his dysphoric mood.

Marcus would also be diagnosed with depressive disorder NOS, because he experienced only four symptoms of depression.

Adjustment Disorder with Depressed Mood

If sadness, irritability, tearfulness, or hopelessness start within three months of the onset of a significant source of stress, and if none of the other mood disorders fit, the appropriate diagnosis may be adjustment disorder with depressed mood. Ten-year-old Shauna had always been a good student, had several close friends, and had gotten along well at home. After her family moved out of state, however, she began crying frequently, seemed very sad, and was convinced that she would never make friends in her new school. After about a month, things began to get better. She started making friends, which made her feel more comfortable in her new school, and her typically sunny disposition reappeared. The diagnosis of an adjustment disorder assumes that there is some difficult situation that requires significant adjustment. If depressive symptoms do not get better when the source of stress goes away or its consequences are removed (within six months), then the diagnosis is changed to an appropriate mood disorder (e.g., MDD or depressive disorder NOS).

Bipolar I Disorder

Bipolar disorder occurs when mania alternates with depression or when manic and depressed symptoms occur simultaneously (called a *mixed episode*). Bipolar I is diagnosed if the mood elevation is severe and if at least three other symptoms of mania occur (four other symptoms are required if the mood is irritable) and if these mood changes last for at least one week. Bipolar I disorder is referred to as *rapid cycling* if four or more manic episodes occur during a one-year period. This criterion differs significantly for children. In children, an ultradian or continuous cycling pattern is more likely (see discussion of bipolar disorder NOS).

BIPOLAR I DISORDER

A. Manic mood (lasting for at least one week):
1. elevated
2. expansive
3. irritable

B. Three (four if irritable mood) of:
1. grandiosity
2. decreased need for sleep
3. increased talking (volume, speed, amount)
4. racing thoughts
5. distractibility
6. increased activity/agitation
7. foolish/reckless behavior (this includes increased interest in sex or hypersexual behavior)

Bipolar II Disorder

Bipolar II involves elevated mood that is clearly "out of character" and behavior that is noted by others but not severe enough to be called manic. When thirteen-year-old Keisha, for example, started making plans faster than her fellow eighth-grade dance committee members could follow, her teachers described her as "supercharged," and one of her teachers had to pull her aside to suggest that she slow down. Keisha's irritable response was totally out of character for her, and her elevated mood, though it could have been attributed to excitement about the upcoming dance, could be viewed as a manic symptom because it was beginning to interfere with her peer relations and had led her to behave inappropriately. BP II can cause significant problems but is easily misdiagnosed or ignored because the symptoms are not extreme. It's important to remember that even moderate symptoms can and should be treated when they are causing impairment or dysfunction.

Cyclothymia

Cyclothymia involves continuous cycling between less severe highs and lows (meaning that no major depressive episodes and no manic episodes occur) over at least one year. This is a chronic condition, meaning that the cycling occurs continuously with very little symptom-free time. These symptoms cause disruption and can be difficult to diagnose. Parents and clinicians should decide together how this should be treated.

Griffin is fourteen and has just begun high school. His mother has described him as having been "moody" since he was young. When he's up, he is bubbly and highly energetic, does well in school, and gets along well with family members. He has lots of ideas and wants to start new projects and activities. When he's down, he's grumpy and hard to get along with at home and tends to isolate himself from others. During elementary school Griffin had a group of friends whom he had known since preschool and who accepted his quirky ups and downs. Once they started middle school, the group separated. Since then, Griffin has struggled socially.

BIPOLAR II DISORDER

A. Hypomanic mood (lasting four to seven days):
   1. elevated
   2. expansive
   3. irritable (hypomania alternating with depression)

B. Three (four if irritable mood) of:
   1. grandiosity
   2. decreased need for sleep
   3. increased talking (volume, speed, amount)
   4. racing thoughts
   5. distractibility
   6. increased activity/agitation
   7. foolish/reckless behavior, including increased interest in sex or hypersexual behavior

Bipolar Disorder Not Otherwise Specified

Since DSM-IV was published in 1994, we have learned a lot about bipolar disorder in children. Barbara Geller and her colleagues at Washington University have conducted extensive research that has confirmed that children tend to display a rapid-cycling picture and, in particular, a continuous cycling pattern. When continuous cycling occurs, manic symptoms occur (elated, highly irritable, or expansive mood along with racing thoughts, grandiose behavior, decreased need for sleep, increased interest in sex), but the episodes are much shorter. For continuous cycling to be diagnosed, these symptoms must occur for at least four hours a day.

Eleven-year-old Donnie has been having more and more trouble functioning at home and at school. He describes himself as "always going up and going down." His mother says she never knows what she is going to get: sometimes he is "high as a kite," laughing and giggling constantly, and at other times he is angry and explosive and prone to long rages. When high—usually two or three times a day, for thirty to ninety minutes at a time—Donnie makes comments about wanting to French kiss his mother and sister, runs through the house screaming at the top of his lungs, talks constantly, and jumps from topic to topic. His rages also last from thirty to ninety minutes and occur at least once but sometimes twice a day. During rages he can become destructive or violent.

Donnie would be diagnosed with BP-NOS, as would a child who demonstrates a significantly elevated mood at times but does not fit the criteria for BP I, BP II, or cyclothymia.

Seasonal Patterns

In some cases, the symptoms of depression or bipolar disorder follow a seasonal pattern. The most common seasonal patterns are the worsening of depressive symptoms in the fall and winter, followed by a return to normal mood, or an "overflow" into hypomania or mania, in the spring and summer. The depressive symptoms that occur in the fall and winter are due to the reduced amount of sunlight available. This seasonal pattern of depression is often accompanied by increased sleep and appetite, carbohydrate craving, and decreased activity. In the springtime, as sunshine returns, life also returns to normal (although, some experience a conversion to mania or hypomania). Phototherapy can be very helpful in managing seasonal patterns; that is discussed further in Chapter 5.

Co-Occurring Disorders

We have just described for you the different ways in which symptoms of mood disorders can occur in children (and adults). Unfortunately, the story is usually somewhat more complex, because childhood mood disorders are often accompanied by co-occurring (or *comorbid*) disorders. Between 40 and 80 percent of children with mood disorders have at least one co-occurring condition. Rates are particularly high among children with early-onset bipolar disorder.

To help you sort out mood symptoms from symptoms of co-occurring disorders, we review commonly co-occurring conditions and how they appear in children with mood disorders. In some cases, treatment for the mood disorder will alleviate the co-occurring symptoms (e.g., antidepressants often reduce anxiety). In other cases, different interventions will be needed to address the co-occurring problem. (You'll learn more about treatment in Chapters 5, 6, and 7.) A thorough evaluation can reveal which, if any, co-occurring disorders your child has. Co-occurring disorders can be grouped into several categories: behavior, anxiety, eating, developmental, and elimination disorders.

BEHAVIOR DISORDERS

Behavior disorders, which co-occur at a high rate with childhood mood disorders, include attention-deficit/hyperactivity disorder (ADHD), oppositional defiant disorder (ODD), conduct disorder, tic disorders, Tourette's disorder, and substance use and abuse disorders. Janet Wozniak and Joseph Biederman and their colleagues at Massachusetts General Hospital found that among a group of children who met criteria for mania, 98 percent also met criteria for co-occurring ADHD (this is not true in reverse—in a group of children with ADHD there is not a high rate of co-occurring mania).

Attention-Deficit/Hyperactivity Disorder. You might notice that some symptoms of ADHD sound very much like symptoms of mania. Because the hallmark of ADHD is difficulty maintaining attention and staying focused appropriately, these symptoms can be difficult to separate from the distractibility of mania or the concentration problems often found in depression. The differences are that ADHD is present by age seven and that symptoms are displayed in a relatively constant fashion, unless treatment (medication and behavioral/environmental management) is in place. The attentional problems associated with mood disorders come and go with mood changes.

Oppositional Defiant Disorder. The hallmark of oppositional defiant disorder (ODD) is a pattern of negative, hostile, and defiant behavior. Accompanying this negativity is a tendency to avoid responsibility and see others as responsible for any problems that occur.

Morgan is nine, and it seems to her parents that she has been arguing and defying them ever since she learned to talk. Six months ago she

ATTENTION-DEFICIT/ HYPERACTIVITY DISORDER

To meet criteria for this diagnosis, some symptoms that cause problems must have started by age seven. If symptoms of inattention are predominant, the diagnosis is ADHD, inattentive type. If hyperactive and impulsive symptoms predominate, the diagnosis is ADHD, hyperactive–impulsive type. If six or more symptoms of inattention and of hyperactivity–impulsivity are present, the diagnosis is ADHD, combined type.

A. Inattention (six or more):
1. makes careless mistakes
2. has difficulty paying attention to school or play tasks
3. doesn't seem to listen
4. doesn't finish tasks
5. has difficulty organizing
6. avoids or dislikes schoolwork or homework
7. loses things
8. is easily distracted
9. is forgetful in daily activities

B. Hyperactivity–impulsivity (six or more):
1. fidgets or squirms
2. fails to stay in seat when it is required
3. runs or climbs excessively
4. has difficulty playing quietly
5. is often "on the go" or acts as if "driven by a motor"
6. talks excessively
7. blurts out answers
8. has difficulty waiting for turn
9. interrupts or intrudes on others

developed an irritable mood that wouldn't go away, began to have difficulty sleeping at night, started picking at rather than eating her food, and began complaining almost constantly about being bored. Morgan began taking an antidepressant and gradually became less irritable, started sleeping better, regained her appetite, and started finding things she enjoyed doing again. However, Morgan continued to insist on always having her way, to argue about anything under the sun, and to blame others for any problem she encountered.

In Morgan's case, the mood symptoms improved with medication, but the co-occurring oppositional and defiant behavior needed to be dealt with through therapy and a change in parenting strategies. Morgan's therapist helped her begin to take responsibility for her behavior and helped her parents carefully pick their battles and learn to hold Morgan accountable for her behavior. Gradually, Morgan began getting along better in the family—following simple family rules without arguing and accepting responsibility for her behavior—although glimpses of Morgan's "You can't boss me around!" attitude linger, especially when she is hungry, tired, or overstimulated.

ODD can occur along with a mood disorder. In some cases, the symptoms are actually part of the mood disorder, and they disappear when the mood disorder is treated, as happened with ten-year-old Sean. Sean is typically agreeable and has a close relationship with his mother. Over the past two months, he began refusing to do things he was asked to do and cursed angrily at his mother when she made suggestions or enforced limits such as his bedtime. It began to feel to Sean's mother as though everything was a fight with him. At the same time, Sean began sleeping two hours less than usual at night, at times was excessively giddy and silly, talked nonstop, and seemed to be supercharged, running around the house at breakneck speed. His mother became fearful that her sweet, loving boy was gone. After a particularly bad afternoon during which Sean cursed and screamed and then threw a pair of scissors at her, his mother called Sean's pediatrician. His pediatrician referred Sean to a psychologist, who did a thorough evaluation, diagnosed Sean with bipolar disorder, and referred him for a medication evaluation. Treatment with a mood stabilizer helped to stabilize Sean's mood, and his hostility and defiance went away as well.

Conduct Disorder. Children and adolescents with conduct disorder show a pattern of behavior that violates the rights of others or the rules of our society. These children repetitively hurt or threaten to hurt people or animals, damage or destroy property, steal or manipulate others, or break important rules. When conduct disorder occurs along with a mood disorder, it can make treatment planning challenging.

Curtis is fourteen and is typically sullen. He hangs around with a group of older teens and doesn't spend any time with kids his own age. Curtis has lost interest in all of the activities that he used to enjoy, including baseball, basketball, and soccer. Although his mother makes sure that he gets to school every day, he sometimes skips classes and rarely does any of the work assigned. Curtis has gotten in many fights at school, and on one occasion he hit a child so hard that he broke his jaw. Despite his mother's attempts to curb this behavior, Curtis frequently starts fires in his room and in the backyard.

After several months of therapy and medication (Curtis took his antidepressant only occasionally, despite reminders from his mother), his mother made the difficult decision to call the police after Curtis hurt his younger brother for no particular reason. After a court appearance, Curtis was placed on probation. With the probation officer's supervision, Curtis began taking his medication. He also attended an after-school program for at-risk youth and began attending mandated family therapy with his mother and brother. Slowly, Curtis's behavior and mood began to improve.

Curtis's mother had to make a difficult decision. The resources of the mental health system were not able to provide enough support for Curtis. To get Curtis the help he needed, she had to go through the juvenile justice system. As a parent of a child or adolescent with a mood disorder, you will need all of the resources available to you. This may require considerable creativity on your part or may cause you to have to do difficult things, such as involving the court system or local law enforcement.

Conduct disorder is diagnosed only if the problems have occurred for at least twelve months and if at least one significant problem has occurred during the past six months. As with ODD, in some cases the conduct problems go away once the mood disorder symptoms are resolved. These situations highlight the need to diagnose the mood disorder and begin treatment.

In addition to severe daily rages, ten-year-old Breanna has started fights at school, injured the family dog, broke many items that did not belong to her, and generally refused to follow rules at home and school. After six months of increasingly disruptive behavior, she was evaluated and diagnosed with bipolar disorder and conduct disorder. She was started on a mood stabilizer, and after several dose adjustments and the addition of a second mood stabilizer, Breanna's mood improved significantly. As her mood stabilized, her behavior also improved. Breanna was once again able to follow rules and to respond to strong emotions without lashing out at those around her.

Tic Disorders. Tic disorders can range from a single transient tic (e.g., lip licking that lasts from four weeks to twelve months) to Tourette's disorder, which involves multiple motor tics (e.g., blinking, shrugging, grimacing) and one or more vocal tics (e.g., throat clearing, repetitive noises). Tic disorders most commonly co-occur with ADHD and obsessive–compulsive disorder but also co-occur with mood disorders. In addition, some medications, particularly stimulant medications, can cause or exacerbate tics.

Substance Use Disorders. Substance use disorders are common among adolescents with mood disorders, with rates as high as 14 percent. In addition to complicating treatment and potentially worsening the course of illness, substance use can mimic mood disorder symptoms. Fifteen-year-old Rachel was diagnosed with bipolar disorder a year ago and has done very well on Depakote. Recently, however, her parents have become more and more concerned about the friends Rachel is choosing. They have tried not to be judgmental about the many body piercings they've noticed, but Rachel has gone from studying with her old friends to hanging out in her room listening to loud music with her new friends. To make matters worse, she has gone from getting A's and B's to getting C's and D's. One afternoon she came home later than usual and was extremely giggly and silly for a couple of hours. Her parents, terrified that the cycling they had lived with previously was beginning again, called Rachel's psychologist. Rachel met alone with her therapist and came clean: She had been smoking marijuana a few times per week for the past several months. On the day that her behavior had been so odd, she had gotten high with her friends after school. Rachel told her therapist that she had felt that things were spiraling out of control. Initially, the marijuana made Rachel feel more calm. Over time, however, getting high had only made Rachel feel more out of control.

It is common for teens to try drugs and alcohol as ways of managing their negative moods. Cigarettes are particularly common. Kendra is sixteen and doesn't remember a time when people and things didn't get on her nerves all the time. She finds that smoking a cigarette when things are really getting to her helps her to stay calm and that smoking helps her feel like she fits in. However, now that Kendra has been smoking for a while, she gets crankier than ever when she can't smoke. Kendra started out smoking one or two cigarettes a day and before she knew it was smoking more than half a pack a day.

Although some drugs can seem to help initially, in most cases they worsen problems in the long run. Although teens often don't realize it, alcohol makes you more depressed. Drugs such as Ecstasy, amphetamines, cocaine, and any of a long list of illegal drugs can cause significant problems for adolescents with mood disorders. In addition to causing mood-disorder-like symptoms and worsening behavior, drugs of abuse may interact with prescribed medications and cause significant complications. Depending on the drug and the amount, drug use can cause permanent damage to the brain or other organs.

ANXIETY DISORDERS

Anxiety disorders are very common among children and adolescents with depression and bipolar disorder. These disorders include separation anxiety disorder, generalized anxiety disorder, specific phobias, obsessive–compulsive disorder, social phobia, panic disorder, and post-traumatic stress disorders.

Separation Anxiety Disorder. Although separation anxiety is a part of normal development in babies and young children, it typically subsides as a child learns that his or her parents always return. Separation anxiety becomes a disorder when it is not developmentally appropriate (e.g., a twelve-year-old who will not go to a sleepover party because she does not want to leave her mother) or is excessive (e.g., a five-year-old who cries and screams upon being dropped off at kindergarten after she has attended school for four months and has received consistent support from teachers and classmates). Separation anxiety disorder also frequently involves worry about losing, or about harm coming to, parents or guardians. In some cases the child fears kidnapping or other harm coming to herself if she is away from parents. Sometimes the anxiety leads to reluctance or refusal to go to school, often with accompanying complaints about physical ailments (e.g., headaches, stomachaches). Separation anxiety disorder is not diagnosed unless it has continued for at least four weeks.

Generalized Anxiety Disorder. The child with generalized anxiety disorder (GAD) is a worrier. The worry can be about any number of events or activities, such as next week's math test, a story he heard on the news, or getting into college (at age twelve). The worry is excessive and causes considerable problems in daily life because much time is spent worrying, resulting in parents spending lots of time trying to soothe and reassure the child. The worrying causes other problems, such as restlessness, difficulty falling asleep, muscle tension, or fatigue. GAD is not diagnosed unless the problem has continued for at least six months.

Specific Phobia. Specific phobia refers to an extreme fear of a particular object or situation, such as a fear of snakes, flying, or heights. For a phobia to be diagnosed, the fear must be so intense that it causes problems, such as refusing to go outside to play with friends because there might be spiders in the yard or resisting a family vacation due to a fear of flying. In response to the feared object or situation, the child becomes extremely anxious and does things such as crying, having a tantrum, freezing, or clinging to a parent. If at all possible, the child avoids the object or situation. Needle phobia can cause difficulty for children recommended for mood stabilizer therapy, as those medicines require ongoing blood draws to monitor safety and efficacy of treatment.

Obsessive–Compulsive Disorder. As the name implies, two types of symptoms occur in obsessive–compulsive disorder (OCD)—obsessive thoughts and compulsive behaviors. Obsessive thoughts tend to be disturbing to the child and cause significant anxiety and distress. Common obsessions include fear of contamination (for example, fear that touching objects will result in getting ill), a need for order (for example, becoming distressed if objects are not placed in a particular order), and repeated doubts (for example, fear that his or her actions have resulted in someone's getting hurt). Compulsions can be repeated behaviors such as hand washing, putting objects in order, or checking repeatedly or mental acts such as counting or repeating words or phrases silently. Compulsions are often a response to disturbing obsessive thoughts and serve as a way to temporarily reduce feelings of anxiety. For example, a boy experiencing a fear of contamination from touching a wall might wash his hands repeatedly, or a girl experiencing obsessive thoughts about her belongings being in order might compulsively lay all of her toys out on the floor in a particular order, then become very upset anytime her mother tries to put them away. Obsessions or compulsions take up a considerable amount of time—an hour or more per day—and disrupt normal routines.

Ten-year-old Ellen gets up at 6:00 A.M. every day and is never ready when the bus comes at 8:15 A.M. She spends up to an hour in the shower washing and carefully rinsing, and she will often get back in the shower if she comes in contact with anything other than her towel for fear that she has gotten dirty again. Once she finally gets her clothes on, she will often change clothes repeatedly, fearing that her outfit has been contaminated. Most days her mother ends up driving her to school, and she is often late.

Social Phobia. Children with social phobia do well in familiar or comfortable social situations (e.g., when playing with a close friend) but experience intense anxiety when asked to perform (e.g., a child who refuses to read in front of the class despite good reading skills, thereby lowering his grade on a project he really enjoyed preparing) or enter an unfamiliar situation. This phobia can prevent a child from participating in after-school activities, hanging out with peers on the weekend, or applying for a part-time job. Often the underlying fear is of being embarrassed or humiliated.

Panic Disorder. A panic attack is an episode of intense fear or discomfort involving a number of different physical symptoms (e.g., pounding heart, sweating, shaking, shortness of breath, feeling like one is choking, chest pain, nausea, dizziness, fear of losing control, fear of dying, numbness or tingling, chills or hot flashes). Panic disorder occurs when a child has frequent panic attacks, as well as significant worrying about another attack occurring. Panic disorder can be accompanied by a fear of leaving home. This anxiety disorder can cause serious problems for children because it can lead to refusals to leave home, attend school, and engage in social activities.

Stress Disorders. Acute stress disorder (ASD) and posttraumatic stress disorder (PTSD) can occur when a child has experienced or witnessed a life-threatening event or an event that significantly undermines a sense of security. Symptoms of ASD and PTSD are nearly the same, although the time course is different. ASD occurs within a month after the traumatic event has occurred; PTSD occurs anytime after the first month posttrauma. ASD and PTSD involve persistent reexperiencing of the event (e.g., intrusive thoughts, images, dreams), avoidance of reminders about the event (e.g., avoiding discussions or places that bring up the event), and increased arousal (e.g., difficulty falling asleep, hypervigilance). ASD also includes what are called *dissociative symptoms,* meaning that the person feels "detached"—from his or her emotions, surroundings, or even memory of the traumatic event. Children can feel awkward or fearful about some events that can cause stress disorders, such as inappropriate fondling from an adult relative or physical fighting between parents, so a careful, sensitive evaluation for the presence or absence of stress disorders is important when completing a comprehensive evaluation.

EATING DISORDERS

Many children with mood disorders experience an increase or decrease in appetite. This can be a symptom of the mood disorder or a side effect of medication. (Unfortunately, many of the mood stabilizers lead to weight gain—we talk more about this in Chapter 6, when we review pharmacological treatments and the management of side effects.)

Weight loss might be due to a mood disorder, to some other health condition, or to anorexia. Anorexia is diagnosed when severe weight loss occurs along with a preoccupation with body image. A child or adolescent with anorexia sees herself as overweight despite being within normal limits or underweight. This child is different from a child who does not eat simply because his appetite is gone due to a medical condition or medication side effect.

A child with bulimia also is preoccupied with concerns about body image. However, a child with bulimia eats large amounts of food in one sitting (for example, an entire package of crackers or cookies) and then finds ways to rid the body of the calories (vomiting, laxative misuse, excessive exercise).

Childhood obesity is a significant public health problem. Overeating and underactivity are the primary culprits, along with poor eating habits. Eating as a maladaptive way to soothe difficult emotions (such as those associated with depression and anxiety), as well as the lethargy that often occurs in depression, can contribute to obesity. In Chapter 9, when we identify methods children can use to manage their emotions, especially anger, you will notice we talk a lot about physical outlets. It is important for all children to be physically active, but for children wrestling with difficult and overwhelming feelings, physical activity can become part of the solution.

DEVELOPMENTAL DISORDERS

This term refers to problems in cognitive development, such as mental retardation and learning disorders, or in social development, such as Asperger's disorder. Children with developmental disabilities can develop mood disorders, and children with mood disorders have a high rate of learning disorders and other developmental problems.

Learning Disorders. For children with mood disorders, school can be challenging. The stress of performing academically and negotiating peer relationships can be very taxing. When a child with a mood disorder also has a learning disorder (also known as a learning disability), school becomes even more stressful. A learning disability is diagnosed when performance in a specific academic area (reading, writing, arithmetic, speech/language) is far below what would be expected based on a child's intelligence. We suspect learning disabilities when a child seems bright but really struggles with some or all parts of school. For example, a child who reads and understands books at or beyond her age level but really resists and struggles with any writing assignment may have a writing disorder. Or the child who is great at math but has a difficult time reading may have a reading disorder. These disorders are diagnosed through intelligence and academic testing. This testing is provided through your child's public school at no cost to you or by a private psychologist. In some cases this testing is covered by insurance, but in many cases it is not. If your child seems to be struggling in certain areas or seems to resist some parts of his schoolwork, you might suspect that a learning disability is getting in your child's way. Estimates vary but suggest that learning disabilities may occur in one-fourth to one-half of children and adolescents with mood disorders. In particular, problems with math are very common for children and teens with bipolar disorder.

Reading, writing, and math learning disabilities are frequently diagnosed and are addressed by providing academic assistance. Some children are very successful academically but struggle in a different domain—nonverbal communication. This is referred to as a nonverbal learning disability (NLD). NLD can severely affect a child's peer and family relationships. A child with a nonverbal learning disability has significantly stronger verbal abilities than nonverbal or visual–spatial abilities. These latter skills are relied on heavily when interpreting social cues, using humor, and judging interpersonal space.

Dante is ten years old and in fourth grade. At the beginning of the school year, he was very sad and cried easily. As a result his classmates avoided him. After starting treatment, his mood improved, but he continued to have difficulty getting along with his classmates despite efforts by his teacher to get him better integrated into the class. His parents were very concerned and requested a meeting with the teacher. During this meeting the teacher described her observations of Dante on the playground. She had noticed that he either stayed to himself or tried awkwardly to enter games. Rather than ask the children if he could join a game, he would just walk up and start bouncing a ball in the middle of their game. The children thus became irritated with him. When the teacher had talked to Dante about it, he seemed to know what he should say, but he never seemed to know how or when to say it. His teacher has been concerned that Dante does not seem to be aware of the nonverbal messages that he sends to others. When children do try to approach him, Dante often behaves in a way that puts other children off. When the teacher tries to talk to Dante about this behavior, he seems unaware of what he has done (for example, turning his back when a child approaches him or talking in a rude tone of voice). Whenever Dante has the chance, he stays in from recess to sit and read a book or do things for his teacher. She noted that Dante is a good student but that writing is very challenging for him. His writing is almost impossible to read, and because of how difficult it is for him to write, he tends to write very little.

Dante is unable to read the body language of his classmates to figure out how and when to enter games. He also has a common problem associated with nonverbal learning disabilities, namely, dysgraphia, or a specific difficulty in writing. Nonverbal learning disabilities are identified through testing and through careful observation. They need to be addressed through therapy and careful management at school and at home, including practicing and drawing attention to reading and conveying body language.

Asperger's Disorder. In this developmental disorder, social development is the primary problem. Children, adolescents, and adults with this disorder have significant problems with social interaction and have patterns of behavior and interests that tend to be repetitive or unusual. Asperger's disorder affects functioning in all settings because it involves difficulty interacting with others. Children with Asperger's disorder often are most comfortable with family members who have learned to accommodate their unusual behavior. Peer relationships tend to be particularly challenging.

Five-year-old Kevin was brought to his pediatrician at age four because of increasing problems getting along in preschool and tantrums that were increasing in intensity. His preschool teachers were finding it very difficult to integrate Kevin into the class because he would fixate on a particular toy and then want to spend the entire day focused on that one toy. For example, one day Kevin wanted to play only with the blocks, but he did not want to build with them—he wanted to look at their angles and sort them into piles of matching blocks. This frustrated the other children, who wanted to build a castle. When his teachers intervened, Kevin began to cry and was inconsolable until his mother came to pick him up an hour later. Despite being at his preschool for over a year, Kevin has not made any friends (although the other children have tried to engage him) and tends to avoid eye contact and isolate himself. Kevin has told his mother he simply isn't interested in the other children's "boring" games and that none of them are as good at matching blocks as he is. At home, Kevin has periods of being sad and withdrawn. His pediatrician has referred him for an evaluation by a psychologist to assess both for Asperger's disorder and for depression.

ELIMINATION DISORDERS

Continuing to have bowel accidents (encopresis) and bladder accidents (enuresis) is also relatively common among children with mood disorders. Physical causes for these problems should always be ruled out by your child's primary care physician. Some children begin to wet themselves as a side effect of medication (usually lithium), as they are more thirsty while on the medicine and tend to drink more. This is an unpleasant side effect, but two effective treatments are available—DDAVP, a nasal spray, or a pager/buzzer system that behaviorally trains the body to wake at night before the child has an accident. (See Resources at the end of this book for information on how to order a pager/buzzer system.)

PSYCHOTIC SYMPTOMS

It is particularly frightening to watch a child experience psychotic symptoms, which are not uncommon in children with severe mood episodes. It is very important to remember: *This is not schizophrenia.* A large percentage of children with bipolar disorder (60 percent in a recent study by Barbara Geller and her colleagues at Washington University) and children with severe episodes of depression experience hallucinations (hearing voices, seeing things, and sometimes smelling or feeling things), delusions (believing she is receiving special messages or has special powers, or other unusual thoughts or ideas). These symptoms occur when mood symptoms are severe. Importantly, they go away when the mood disorder is treated.

During the evaluation process, both your child's mood disorder and his co-occurring disorders should be identified. In some cases, the co-occurring disorders will be left as "rule-outs," so your clinician can later determine if symptoms of the co-occurring disorder were actually part of the mood disorder (for example, a child who seems to be very defiant and argumentative may have ODD, or these symptoms might abate once the irritability associated with his depression is treated). Sometimes it's difficult to sort out mood disorder symptoms from those of a co-occurring disorder. In these cases, starting treatment for the mood disorder and seeing what remains once the mood disorder remits is the only way to separate mood symptoms from co-occurring disorders.

If this all sounds confusing to you, rest assured that you are not alone. Most parents of children with mood disorders grapple not only with mood symptoms but also with one or more of the co-occurring disorders we described here.

What Do I Do If Things Don't Go the Way I Expected?

Let's suppose you have waited six weeks to get an evaluation (after trying for three weeks to get a referral). You are at your wits' end, and your child seems to be getting worse by the day. You have prepared well for the evaluation—kept records of your child's moods, written down your questions, and arranged for both you and your spouse to be off work the afternoon of the evaluation. You have all of your bases covered. The clinician meets with you and your spouse, takes a quick look at the notes you prepared, and meets alone with your child. She then meets again with you and your spouse and asks about conflict at home and how you set limits for your son or daughter. She doesn't seem to be focusing on the issue you came to address. You begin to feel uncomfortable. This was not the discussion you had expected. You begin to wonder whether the clinician believed or even listened to anything you said about your child's moods and behavior. What do you do? Hang in there a little while longer. Sometimes clinicians will go after information in a different way from what you have organized in your head.

Also, it's common for parents to feel a range of emotions following an initial evaluation. If you have questions about how the initial evaluation went, ask them at your first follow-up appointment. If you continue to feel uncomfortable about how things are going, or if the clinician seems to be avoiding your questions or discounting your input, don't ignore your gut. Share your concerns with the clinician. If that is not successful, get a second opinion. You should also get a second opinion if the clinician tells you that children cannot get mood disorders; if that happens, he or she is definitely not the "expert" that you want and need.

Part II

Treatment

Getting an accurate diagnosis of your child's mood problems, along with any co-occurring disorders, is important groundwork for effective treatment of your child. In our work with families we have found, however, that educated consumers often benefit the most from treatment. So in the following chapters we explain what you can expect as you navigate through your child's treatment process. Whether you are new to treatment or have experience with another family member's treatment, knowing what to expect will help you use your resources well.

Chapter 5 presents the "big picture"—some general principles to guide you through the treatment process, plus an overview of different types of treatment. In Chapter 6 we help you think about the benefits and costs of medications so you can make thoughtful decisions about medications for your child. We introduce you to commonly prescribed medications and describe how you can monitor the efficacy of the treatment and manage any side effects. In Chapter 7 we describe the role of psychotherapy in children's mood disorders so you can work with your child's doctor in devising the best possible combination of interventions for your unique child.

5 | Getting the Big Picture

There's no question that treating mood disorders in children (and in adults, for that matter) can be complicated. As you've learned, it's not easy to sort out a child's mood problems, and many children end up diagnosed with more than one disorder. Even the simplest cases may require trial and error to arrive at the best possible treatment plan. This chapter helps you enter the treatment process with a strong foundation: some principles to keep in mind, a basic knowledge of the treatment options available, and an understanding of what treatment often looks like for the different mood disorders.

Rules to Live By

In any complicated situation—and parenting a child with a mood disorder certainly qualifies—having a sense of the big picture can make dealing with the many details much easier down the road. As you access care and follow through with treatment for your child, you'll be making many decisions, evaluating the decisions made by others in the name of helping your child, and interacting with a variety of providers. The following guiding principles will help you stay focused on your goals for your child and on the unavoidable realities of mood disorders.

Mood Disorders Are Complicated

The complexity of childhood mood disorders means that the best way to address them *usually* involves more than one kind of intervention. Treatment components may include: individual therapy, family therapy, medications, parent guidance, school-based interventions, group therapy, light therapy, environmental adaptations, inpatient treatment, partial hospitalization, therapeutic boarding schools, electroconvulsive therapy (in severe, difficult-to-treat cases), and/or alternative living arrangements. In addition, to best help your child, treatment might include the diagnosis and treatment of other family members, including parents and siblings. Setting your expectations for a multitiered approach will make it easier for you to accommodate and adapt to the different recommendations you receive.

Cost–Benefit Analyses Are Key

All treatments have costs, as well as benefits. There's the monetary cost, of course, but there are also nonfinancial costs, such as the risk of medication side effects, administration difficulties (the needle phobia mentioned in Chapter 4, for one), the scheduling hassles associated with attending regular therapy sessions thirty-five minutes or more away from home, the need to find child care for your other children during these appointments, or the time you have to take off from work to attend your child's sessions. Part of your job as your child's advocate is to decide whether the *cost* of a treatment component is worth its potential *benefit* (for example, better coping skills, improved mood, and better quality of life for you, your child, and your family). Don't be embarrassed to talk this through with your child's primary clinician. For example, if a therapist recommends a specialized summer camp program and you don't think you can afford the tuition, say so. There may be scholarships that would make the camp an option for your family. Similarly, some medications are more costly than others. If paying the difference between two similar medications is a hardship for you, don't hesitate to share this concern with your prescribing physician. All families are different, and if you don't share this sort of input with your clinician, she might make treatment recommendations that are not feasible or that come at an extremely high personal price for your family. Or your clinician might wonder why you don't follow through with the excellent advice he is providing you.

Timing Is Everything

Because your growing child is a moving target, the treatment needed now is not necessarily the treatment that will be needed six months down the road. Your job is to work together with your treatment providers to determine what components of care are most appropriate for your child at any point in time. For example, you may need to decide when to try medication or when help at school is needed. For a child who is evaluated at age four, the cost of trying medication might be too high until other interventions, such as parent guidance, have been tried first. However, by age six, if symptoms have worsened and problems at school and with peers are increasing, beginning a medication trial may be in order. Deciding when to try medication can be particularly difficult, especially for parents of young children. We explore this decision-making process more thoroughly in Chapter 6.

You Have to Count Your "Piles"

As you learned in Chapter 4, children's mood disorders often come with associated problems or co-occurring disorders. Families we've worked with have found it helpful to think about their problems as falling into separate "piles." For example, ten-year-old Amy becomes overly excited, very silly, very easily angered, and makes dangerous or inappropriate choices (she recently bit another child while they were arguing about what game to play during recess). In addition, she worries about everything and is often uncomfortable in group situations, which causes her to become hyperactive and silly to relieve her discomfort. On top of those problems, she has difficulty focusing on her schoolwork. All of this felt overwhelming to both Amy and her mother.

Following an evaluation by a psychiatrist, Amy was diagnosed with bipolar disorder, and Amy's bipolar symptoms were identified as the first "pile" to address—extreme moods, poor judgment, and hyperactivity. Amy was started on a mood stabilizer and had a terrific response to the medication, her moods leveled out, she stopped making poor choices, and her activity was reduced to a tolerable (though still high) level. This improvement allowed Amy and her mom to focus on her second "pile"— anxiety. Amy's persistent worrying and extreme social discomfort were addressed effectively through individual therapy, in which Amy learned techniques to manage her anxiety, plus being prescribed a low-dose antidepressant.

Now, with the first two piles "swept away," the third pile became clearer. Amy continued to have difficulty staying focused on her schoolwork and was very impulsive—she touched things she shouldn't touch and forgot to think before she acted. Her psychiatrist suggested a trial of a low-dose stimulant. This was quite helpful in simmering down Amy's impulsivity, further reduced her "busy" behavior, and helped Amy stay focused, both during the school day and after school, as she completed her homework.

Thinking in terms of piles can help your child's problems seem more manageable. One pile may be left alone in a corner until other piles are dealt with (typically the mood symptoms come first on the list). At other times, another pile might be swept up and thrown away as it is resolved completely. Each pile involves a different set of problems. It's useful to know how many and what kind of piles you're dealing with so that you can develop a plan for each. Later in this chapter, we follow several children through treatment. You'll see that some piles can be addressed simultaneously, whereas others have to be addressed in sequence.

Can't and Won't Are Not Synonymous

In addition to the set of piles that separate mood from anxiety, behavior, and developmental problems, you may want to think in terms of a "can't" and a "won't" pile. By this we mean that there are some behaviors that your child *can't* control and other behaviors that your child *won't* control. Differentiating "can't" behaviors from "won't" behaviors helps parents remember that the enemy is the mood disorder and that the mood symptoms are beyond the child's control. For example, if your daughter is depressed, she can't help feeling irritable or being unable to fall asleep. If your son is in the middle of a severe manic episode and comes into the kitchen looking all worked up, he can't help flying into a rage when you tell him it's time for dinner and you're having hamburgers. However, if your daughter snaps at you when you ask her to get off the computer then turns around and is sweet as pie to her best friend who calls on the phone fifteen seconds later, she probably could have curbed her tongue with you—that is a "won't" behavior. Likewise, if your son is calmly watching television and you tell him to turn the TV off in five minutes when the show ends and he refuses to do so, this is probably a "won't"— he won't comply with your request.

The challenge for parents is figuring out how to make this distinction. Intuitive parents have taught us a lot. When parents describe "can't" behavior, they use such phrases as, "He gets that wild look in his eyes" or "She's gone." "Won't" behavior is more likely to be depicted as, "She gets that naughty twinkle in her eye, and then she goes for it" or

"He gets a nasty little smile on his face, like 'I don't have to listen to you!'" Think about what you've witnessed with your child, and see if you can start to differentiate between her *can'ts* and *won'ts*.

Learning to make this distinction is important. Not recognizing the *can'ts* is frustrating for you and your child. You will find yourself holding your child accountable for expectations she can't meet, which leads to a sense of failure on her part and yours. On the other hand, not holding children accountable for "won't" behavior can train them to be "little monsters," who, of course, grow bigger and less charming over time.

Usually, mood symptoms have to be treated before you can successfully separate the *can'ts* from the *won'ts*. This is the first step in decreasing the amount of "can't" behavior. "Won't" behavior also needs careful treatment. Unfortunately, "won't" behavior doesn't always go away with medication—but you may find that it slowly begins to melt away as your child learns better coping skills through therapy and as you gradually change communication patterns, rules, and household structure to eliminate it.

Types of Treatment

Mood disorders are biological illnesses—there is either too much or too little of certain chemicals (neurotransmitters) in the brain. Mood disorders are also psychological; patterns of thinking and behavior are disturbed. And mood disorders are social. They are affected by what goes on around them. Treatment, therefore, needs to be *biopsychosocial:* It needs to address all three components.

Keep in mind as you read about the three types of interventions that they are often used in some combination to treat mood disorders. This same biopsychosocial model applies to co-occurring disorders. In some cases, co-occurring problems will be treated in part by mood-disorder treatments. For example, many anxiety disorders and some behavior disorders and eating disorders respond very well to the same medications that are used to treat depression. However, most co-occurring disorders will require some other specialized intervention, such as other medications or psychotherapy, school intervention, or learning to cope with (and sometimes accept) the symptoms of those disorders.

Biological Treatments

MEDICATIONS

Medications can be used very effectively to treat mood disorders. The challenge with medications is to find the right medication or combination of medications, at the right doses and the right administration times, to reduce mood symptoms with the fewest possible side effects. There is no magic formula to determine who will respond best to which medication. Although dosage guidelines may help, there is no surefire way to decide what dose will work best for any particular child. We discuss these issues and the different types of available medications in more detail in Chapter 6.

DIETARY INTERVENTION

Recent research has suggested that some supplements (omega-3 fatty acids and a vitamin–mineral complex called EMpowerplus) might be helpful for treating mood disorders, especially bipolar disorder. Studies conducted with adults have found that taking omega-3 fatty acids can improve short-term outcome for adults with bipolar disorder. Andrew Stoll and his colleagues at McLean Hospital in Massachusetts have shown that omega-3 fatty acids augment the effects of mood stabilizers in adults with bipolar disorder and depression; they increase periods of time without symptoms and improve the course of illness. Although there are no completed studies of the effectiveness of omega-3 fatty acids in children, some studies are under way. (See the Resources at the end of this book for information about omega-3 fatty acids.)

In preliminary research with adults, Bonnie Kaplan and her colleagues at the University of Calgary have shown significant symptom reduction in patients taking the broad-spectrum vitamin–mineral complex called EMpowerplus, as well as a decreased need for medication. Clinical observations in children are promising, and further research is under way. (See the Resources for information about EMpowerplus.)

LIGHT THERAPY

For children whose depressive symptoms worsen during the fall and winter months, use of light therapy is very effective. Light therapy can be used to treat depression that occurs only in the fall and winter months, when there is less natural exposure to light. This may be especially relevant for people living in locations that experience a high number of gray, cloudy days. Light therapy involves sitting in front of a specially designed light box for thirty to forty minutes once or twice a day. (See the Resources for information about seasonal affective disorder and its treatment.)

If your child experiences seasonal depression patterns, moving to a warmer, sunnier climate might improve your child's condition as well. This should be kept in mind when making decisions about where to live, such as in choosing a college for an older adolescent.

ELECTROCONVULSIVE THERAPY (ECT)

In the popular press, electroconvulsive therapy (ECT) has been associated with old-fashioned and cruel treatments for the mentally ill (as was depicted in the film *One Flew Over the Cuckoo's Nest*). Despite the stigma associated with it, ECT continues to be used, very effectively and humanely, for people who experience severe depression that does not respond to medication. It is administered under general anesthesia and involves an electric shock to the brain that causes a seizure. If you were to watch someone as ECT was conducted, you would find it to be very anticlimactic. The individual would appear to be sleeping peacefully with electrodes taped to her head. Only by looking at the monitor would you be able to see that a seizure was occurring. How and why this works is not completely clear, but ECT can be a lifesaver for someone with severe depression who has not improved on many different medications. This type of treatment is used *very* rarely with adolescents and almost never with children.

Psychological Treatments (Therapy)

Different types of therapy have different goals and objectives. Many therapists (usually psychologists or social workers) use a hybrid approach, in which a combination of, for example, individual therapy and parent guidance might occur within each scheduled session. A key element in any type of therapy is that you feel comfortable sharing your feelings and experiences with the therapist. Psychotherapy research has taught us that what professionals call "nonspecific factors" (e.g., whether your therapist is a likable person—warm, genuinely interested in your situation, attentive to your concerns) are very important in terms of favorable outcomes, regardless of the type of therapy being provided.

We discuss goals of therapy in more detail in Chapter 7. Here we provide a brief overview of the different types of therapy.

INDIVIDUAL THERAPY

This type of therapy involves the child or adolescent with the mood disorder working one on one with the therapist. It varies tremendously from therapist to therapist and from child to child. Individual therapy may focus on building coping skills, increasing understanding of symptoms, identifying and building strengths, recognizing and changing negative thoughts and behavior, or strengthening interpersonal skills.

FAMILY THERAPY

This type of therapy involves the child or adolescent and one or more family members. Sometimes the term *conjoint* is used to describe the child working in a session along with one parent. Goals for family therapy might include improving communication and resolving problems.

PARENT GUIDANCE

Mood disorders are complex and can cause many problems in family life. To make matters worse, no life experience can prepare you to raise a child with a mood disorder. Being a "good enough" parent is not necessarily "good enough" to give you the skills to manage your child through these difficult times. Therefore, parent guidance is often an important part of therapy for a child with a mood disorder. The goal of parent guidance is to help parents develop specific strategies that might be helpful for their particular child, as well as to accept the child's illness and develop realistic expectations.

GROUP THERAPY

Group therapy involves several children or adolescents working with one or more therapists simultaneously. The advantages of group therapy include the support that group members provide to one another, the ability of same-age peers to give meaningful feedback to a peer in a way that no adult can, the opportunities for practicing social skills during sessions, and the expediency of teaching skills to several children at one time.

Social or Environmental Interventions

SCHOOL-BASED INTERVENTIONS

Some children with mood disorders will have co-occurring conditions, such as learning and behavior disorders, that require specialized intervention at school. In addition, some mood disorder symptoms affect learning, such that adjustments at school may be necessary, at least on a temporary basis. For example, a child who has been hospitalized for a severe depressive episode may need to begin with home instruction following discharge from the hospital, then progress to attending school part time, then work up to attending school full time with support from a guidance counselor when needed. In Chapter 10, we discuss in much greater detail how to help your child at school.

HOME-BASED INTERVENTIONS

During times of crisis, it may be helpful to have a home-based therapist work with you. The goals of home-based interventions are to equip parents to manage difficult behaviors and to develop plans for managing crises. Crisis management may involve a therapist coming to your home in the midst of the situation. Usually home-based therapists are part of a clinic staff. If you receive intervention from a private psychiatrist or psychologist, you will be less likely to work with a home-based therapist.

RESPITE

When a child requires around-the-clock close supervision and support (as is true of some children with mood disorders), parents burn out quickly. The goal of respite care is to give parents an opportunity to recover. For some families with extensive support networks, respite might be provided by friends or family members. In other situations there may be no one in your social circle who is willing or able to provide respite care for your child. Some agencies provide respite care, but you may have to work hard to find and arrange for those services.

OUT-OF-HOME PLACEMENTS

When a child's behavior at home is unmanageable, out-of-home placement may be necessary. This may mean moving in temporarily or permanently with another family member (especially when conflict between the child and an immediate family member is a serious problem) or placement in a residential treatment program or school. Out-of-home placements usually don't occur unless less restrictive alternatives (e.g., intensive outpatient therapy, short-term hospitalization) have failed.

Funding can be a significant roadblock to out-of-home placement. Insurance may cover some of the cost of a residential treatment program but may provide for only a limited stay. Therapeutic boarding schools can be helpful but are very expensive and usually are not covered by insurance.

Unfortunately, the only way for many families to get access to residential treatment is through public funding. This puts families in the very difficult position of either temporarily signing custody of their child (and therefore clinical decision making) over to the state or county or forgoing much-needed services. Consumer advocacy groups are working hard to change this policy, and the situation may improve in the future, but currently some families are asked to make a heart-wrenching decision if their child cannot be maintained safely within their home.

How Treatment Works for Specific Mood Disorders

All children are different, and appropriate treatment can vary tremendously from child to child and family to family. One factor to keep in mind is that, as your son or daughter continues to develop, his or her treatment will have to evolve, as well. Here's what this might look like in the case of specific mood disorders. Notice the biopsychosocial approach to treatment in the examples that follow.

Major Depressive Disorder

Ann Marie is nine, and her parents are both being treated successfully for anxiety and depression. When Ann Marie began to exhibit depressive symptoms similar to those of her parents, they shared this concern with their family physician, who prescribes their medications. Their doctor agreed to put Ann Marie on medication as long as her parents agreed to schedule an appointment for Ann Marie with a therapist skilled with young children. Ann Marie showed an immediate positive response to the medication. Her eating, sleeping, and concentration at school all improved. Ann Marie's therapist helped Ann Marie understand why she was struggling with peers and helped her develop strategies to increase her social interactions. This helped Ann Marie enjoy recess at school and she began to feel better about herself. She also became more successful at arranging play activities on the weekends with other children. Ann Marie's therapist also coached her parents to stop grilling their daughter every evening about how school had gone, which made Ann Marie uncomfortable, and to focus instead on spending fifteen to twenty minutes in the evening on a fun family activity.

Paul is twelve and miserable! He's in sixth grade and started middle school this year. He cries frequently, spends most of his time alone in his room, and can barely concentrate on his schoolwork. He frequently takes naps and has considerable difficulty getting up in the morning. He has gained fifteen pounds since the beginning of the school year and is beginning to look overweight. In elementary school Paul had a few friends, but his two closest friends went on to private school, and he has not had any success in making new friends.

After Paul's complaints about school became intense, his parents took him to see a psychologist, who learned from Paul that, in addition to finding the workload overwhelming, he'd been bullied by a group of eighth graders. He also learned that Paul hadn't told his parents or teachers about what was bothering him because he had assumed they wouldn't be able to help. Knowing that someone cared about his troubles lifted a huge burden from Paul's shoulders. Paul was diagnosed with depression and was scheduled for psychoeducational testing at school. This identified a reading disability. Paul's parents immediately scheduled a meeting with the school. A plan was developed to address the bullying, which included Paul's working with the therapist on ways he could respond to the bullies, the school principal's addressing the bullies directly, and a safe adult being identified for Paul to go to if the problems recurred. To address the learning disability, Paul was scheduled to spend one period per day with a reading specialist. In addition to this one-on-one work, the reading specialist would help his teacher modify assignments so that they would be more manageable for Paul. His psychologist also suggested that Paul join a twelve-week therapy group focused on social skills. In family sessions, Paul and his parents worked on ways to strengthen their relationships so that Paul would not feel so isolated at home. The family began planning weekly family activities during family meetings, which included Paul's ten-year-old brother. Paul and his parents agreed with the psychologist to reevaluate the need for medication after these other interventions were in place.

Fifteen-year-old Brandon has a history of anxiety, including panic attacks. Following a period of escalating panic attacks, he began to experience increasingly severe depressive symptoms, for which he was prescribed Prozac without any significant improvement. He dropped out of sports and then band and had difficulty attending school. Ultimately, Brandon started to have intense suicidal thoughts and had such difficulty concentrating that he couldn't read a novel, despite having been a straight-A student in the past. Multiple medications were tried, again with little improvement. Brandon started intensive individual therapy with a focus on providing him support, activity planning (using involvement in activities to help manage his mood), anxiety management strategies, and identifying and trying to change thought patterns that perpetuated his depressed feelings. Ultimately Brandon was hospitalized due to suicidal thoughts; he was able to leave the hospital when he felt confident that he would not act on these thoughts. However, Brandon was still very depressed and unable to attend school. Intensive individual and family therapy (at least once per week) was continued while Brandon began home instruction. Eight months later Brandon's improvement was minimal. Following considerable discussion among Brandon, his parents, and their treatment providers, the decision was made to try a series of ECT. After the first two treatments, Brandon began to show some improvement. His ECT was concluded after six treatments. Brandon's mood had improved dramatically. He continued treatment with two atypical antidepressants after ECT ended. Brandon gradually added activities back into his schedule until he had resumed his typical routine. Brandon was able to start the next school year with his peers. He returned to getting straight A's.

Dysthymic Disorder

Eight-year-old Michelle has been unhappy "since birth," according to her mother, Annette. Annette sought therapy for Michelle after talking to her sister-in-law, whose ten-year-old son had had similar problems and made considerable improvement with therapy. When Michelle and Annette initially met with the therapist, Michelle sat in her mother's lap and refused to talk. The therapist assured Annette that this was not unusual. Annette and Michelle continued attending sessions, which were split between individual time for Michelle and parent guidance for Annette. Parent guidance helped Annette begin to separate Michelle's symptoms from her personality (this can be particularly difficult to do when children have dysthymic disorder, as their symptoms have been chronic and can appear to be part of their personality) and to learn new ways of responding to Michelle's irritability. After making little progress over a two-month period, Michelle's therapist suggested a medication consultation. Once she started on medication, Michelle's mood began to improve, and she was more willing to work actively in therapy. Michelle and her therapist developed strategies to improve her peer network and came up with ideas that Michelle could try when she felt sad or irritable, such as playing with her dog or reading a book from her favorite series.

Anthony is sixteen and has been grumpy since puberty. He has begun smoking some marijuana. Although he used to have a large group of friends, Anthony now spends time with only a few friends who, from his parents' perspective, seem to have significant problems. Although he had been a good athlete, Anthony dropped out of sports and is no longer an active member of the drama club. After finding marijuana in his pants pocket while doing the laundry, Anthony's parents sought an evaluation for him. Anthony was diagnosed with dysthymic disorder and substance abuse disorder. Therapy and random drug screening were recommended, in addition to a medication evaluation. Anthony refused to participate in therapy. He also told his parents that he would not take "their" medication and that they shouldn't waste their money on "drugging [him] with pharmaceutical poison." Despite his protests, Anthony's parents began working with the therapist on their own. Parent guidance helped them make some changes in their responses to Anthony's behavior. Aware that they were going to sessions and probably talking about him, Anthony decided that he didn't want "people talking behind my back" and began attending therapy sessions. Although he started the first session with his arms crossed over his chest and a sullen look on his face, Anthony eventually complained that his parents always yell at him and never spend time with him, except to reprimand him and give him lectures. Anthony's parents responded by agreeing to discuss rather than yell, as long as Anthony would listen to what they had to say, and to plan one night a week to go out to dinner or order pizza together. Anthony didn't say much in response to their offer, but a look of satisfaction passed across his face. After several more sessions with similar negotiations, Anthony eventually agreed to a medication evaluation. Ultimately, Anthony began taking an antidepressant. His mood improved significantly, and he began reinitiating some of his previous activities. His parents commented on how much they appreciated having had a "referee" in their therapy sessions to negotiate what otherwise would have felt like "irreconcilable differences."

Bipolar Disorder

Ten-year-old Julia described her mood state as "overstimulated," a term she had probably heard from one of the adults in her life. It turned out she meant a combination of anger, anxiety, excitement, happiness, and frustration. She became anxious and agitated whenever presented with any change in schedule or unexpected event. Although her mother was often able to recognize when Julia needed to leave situations to "de-stimulate," Julia tended to resist her prompts and was having increasing peer problems as a result of emotional crises in the presence of peers and at school. Julia also had some pretty wild schemes. She was sure that she was going to be a movie star and win an Academy Award, so she practiced her acceptance speech daily and frequently dressed up using lots of bright makeup. She often complained that her thoughts "moved faster than the speed of light." She was typically the first to awaken in her family (around 5:00 A.M.) and often the last to fall asleep at night.

Her mother found a clinician on her insurance company's provider list who could evaluate Julia, but she was concerned about the fact that the clinician saw very few children and didn't seem knowledgeable about Julia's kind of difficulties. Fortunately, Julia's mother shared these impressions with her next-door neighbor, a school guidance counselor, who recommended a local child and adolescent psychiatrist with expertise in mood disorders. The psychiatrist diagnosed Julia with bipolar disorder and prescribed a mood stabilizer. After Julia was on a therapeutic level, he added a low-dose antidepressant. The psychiatrist also referred Julia's family to a psychologist experienced in childhood mood disorders. The psychologist initiated individual psychotherapy, alternating with parent guidance. Once Julia's mood was stabilized, co-occurring ADHD was diagnosed and a low-dose stimulant medication was added. Therapy continued throughout this process, and co-occurring problems were also addressed. A psychoeducational evaluation was conducted to explore academic issues and to assist in devising an academic plan. Julia was also referred to a dietician to address weight and food choice issues.

As therapy progressed and Julia got older, her responsibilities in managing her illness and her behavior were increasingly emphasized. Sessions decreased in frequency until Julia saw her psychiatrist only once every six months; her mother was advised to call their psychologist if problems came up that they did not know how to solve on their own or if they noticed signs of relapse (which their psychologist reviewed thoroughly with them in their final regularly scheduled session).

When Julia hit middle school, however, it became increasingly difficult for her to negotiate the complexities of this new, more elaborate social scene. Julia needed more assistance and support in therapy to help her deal with social issues. Because she was so comfortable with her psychologist, Julia was able to "check in" for several sessions until they developed a new "middle school game plan" that gave Julia ideas for how to manage the new stressors of meeting many new kids and teachers, getting used to a new school building, and transferring classrooms. They also designated a new "home base" (the assistant principal's office), where she could go to de-escalate, as this strategy had provided her a strong sense of security while in elementary school.

Andy is eleven. His moods cycle from angry to hyperactive to extremely sad many times a day. His rages are frequent and severe, and he is extremely oppositional and defiant, arguing about almost everything said to him. As Andy became progressively more aggressive during rages, sometimes targeting his four-year-old sister, his behavior at school became increasingly unmanageable, and he was recommended for placement in a severe behavioral handicap (SBH) classroom. He gets into struggles at his mom and step-dad's home as well as at his dad's home, where he spends every other weekend.

After Andy had seen several different therapists, each of whom seemed overwhelmed by Andy's symptoms, his mother, Connie, called her insurance company to get a referral to a child and adolescent psychiatrist. The psychiatrist started Andy on a mood stabilizer, then added an atypical antipsychotic, Risperdal (we discuss the use of atypicals in treating bipolar disorder in more detail in Chapter 6). After reading on the Internet (see the Resources) about the benefits of omega-3 fatty acids for children with bipolar disorder, Connie asked the psychiatrist about this alternative treatment and was encouraged to add the supplement to Andy's regimen. The psychiatrist also referred Andy to a therapist in her office who was well versed in childhood mood disorders. The therapist began working individually with Andy and provided parent guidance to Andy's mother and stepfather. Andy's father also came to several sessions, which helped decrease the friction between the two households over issues regarding the management of Andy's disorder.

After a particularly severe rage during which Andy grabbed a knife and threatened his younger sister, Andy was hospitalized for six days.

During his hospitalization, a second mood stabilizer was added, and Andy was referred for case management. Andy's case manager helped to coordinate his services and saw him regularly at school. She also helped Connie work with the school to optimize his school program. Through a local organization and with Andy's therapist's encouragement, Connie arranged respite care for Andy for four hours every other weekend, when he otherwise would be with her. Although this was not a lot of time, it did allow her and Andy's stepfather to spend special time with Andy's sister and with each other. With the addition of medication, Andy's mood began to stabilize. He still experienced periods of irritability and sadness, but the fluctuations became less dramatic and less frequent.

However, Andy continued to have at least one severe tantrum each day, usually after being asked to do something or to stop doing something. During these tantrums, Andy frequently hit his mother and destroyed property. Again with his therapist's encouragement, Connie called the local police during one of his tantrums. Andy appeared with his parents in front of a family court judge, who ordered him into a youth diversion program that involved working with a probation officer on a weekly basis. Connie was impressed that Andy worked very hard to control his behavior after this occurred, because he didn't want to be sent to the juvenile detention center in his community.

Seasonal Patterns

By November during his junior year, sixteen-year-old Alec had become lethargic, seemed to lose interest in his schoolwork and friends, and wanted to avoid all pressure by sleeping. These behaviors were out of character for him, although in the past Alec had noticed that he had a pattern of slowing down during the middle of the school year. Alec also began to overeat and gained twelve pounds in one month without a comparable gain in height. Over the midwinter school break Alec's mood did not improve substantially. He finally asked his parents if he could see someone to help him with his problems. Alec's family doctor suggested he go to see a psychologist. The psychologist diagnosed Alec with seasonal affective disorder. In addition to some short-term therapy, the psychologist recommended that Alec use a light box. Alec began treatment in early January, and within three weeks he became more invested in friends and schoolwork, lost five pounds, and returned to his typical amount of sleep.

Let's Be Practical

With treatment needs almost guaranteed to change over time, you are most likely to get what you need if you're well prepared. You can help your child and your family best by being aware of what resources your family and your community have to offer and by continuing to be an active partner in the process.

Family Resources

What services does your insurance cover? Which providers are included under your coverage? For therapy to be effective, it needs to occur at regular intervals, such as once a week or once every other week initially; so you need to determine how much your insurance covers and how much you can afford. Some insurance programs cover a percentage of the cost, which may leave you with a significant out-of-pocket expense. Visits to the psychiatrist may be less frequent, but here too you need to know what you can afford. Depending on your primary care physician's comfort level and on the complexity of your child's needs, a pediatrician or family doctor may provide effective medication management.

Community Resources

In addition to knowing what you can afford, you need to know what is available. You may need to become a super sleuth. Ask questions. Your pediatrician or family doctor may be a good place to start. Is there an identi-

---

| **TIPS FOR PARENTS** |

Questions to answer when starting treatment:

1. How much and what treatments does my insurance cover?

2. What is my out-of-pocket cost?

3. Who in my local area is covered?

4. Do I have other resources for getting mental health care?

    a. Does my child qualify for Social Security Insurance (SSI) or Medicaid? (More about that in Chapter 12.)

    b. Can I afford to pay for some services out-of-pocket?

    c. Are there any sources of funding available in my community? (Leave no stone unturned—some notable examples are a special state-administered fund to provide health care and mental health services for adopted children or a fund through the probation department that can pay for short-term, specific interventions.)

fiable expert or specialty clinic for childhood mood disorders in your area? These resources might be based at a local university or hospital. Contact your local consumer-based group, for example, the National Alliance for the Mentally Ill (NAMI), the Mental Health Association (MHA), or the Child and Adolescent Bipolar Foundation for referrals. (See the Resources for ways to contact these organizations.) Your insurance company may also be a good resource. Some insurance programs have care managers who can be helpful in finding appropriate resources.

FAMILY EXERCISE 3: BUILDING YOUR MENTAL HEALTH TEAM

As a good consumer and as your child's advocate, you need to periodically review the services you have and their respective goals then determine what, if anything, you continue to need. Figure 9 shows Julia's mental health team (she's the ten-year-old with bipolar disorder described earlier in this chapter). Look at her example, then diagram your own team on a piece of paper—the members already on board and the types of members you still need. You'll notice that the team includes your child, your family, and your child's school. Each of these team members plays an important role. Your child spends much of his time at school. Therefore, he may need a variety of support services at school (regardless of whether he has any specific learning challenges). And your child is surrounded by family. Small changes or simply increased awareness and understanding can help all family members learn to adapt to the challenges of a mood disorder.

• *Coordinate and clarify roles.* Once you have started the ball rolling, you may need to put some effort in to coordinating services and clarifying roles. By the time Andy, our eleven-year-old with bipolar disorder and ODD, got out of the hospital, he had a psychiatrist, psychologist, probation officer, case manager, and respite care provider. Each person working with Andy had a different, important role in Andy's treatment. The different types of treatment interact. For example, therapy often is more effective when a child is medicated appropriately. Likewise, the prescribing physician will be better equipped to make medication adjustments if he is in communication with your child's therapist.

Roles of treatment providers need to be well defined to ensure that treatment is effective and that services are not redundant. If you are ever unsure about what role a particular provider is playing, ask. Although you may have a case manager assigned to help you, you are ultimately the manager and coordinator of care for your child. For example, Andy's psychiatrist sees him and his mother once a month for thirty minutes (appointment lengths for medication checks usually range from fifteen to thirty minutes). The psychologist sees Andy and his mother, Connie, for fifty minutes every other week (typically twenty minutes with Connie alone, twenty minutes with Andy, and ten minutes with both together). She also stays in close contact

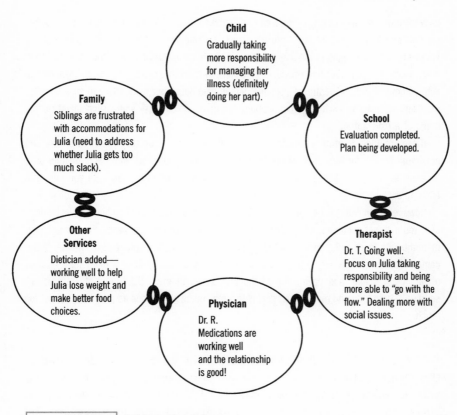

Child
Gradually taking more responsibility for managing her illness (definitely doing her part).

Family
Siblings are frustrated with accommodations for Julia (need to address whether Julia gets too much slack).

School
Evaluation completed. Plan being developed.

Other Services
Dietician added— working well to help Julia lose weight and make better food choices.

Physician
Dr. R. Medications are working well and the relationship is good!

Therapist
Dr. T. Going well. Focus on Julia taking responsibility and being more able to "go with the flow." Dealing more with social issues.

FIGURE 9 | Julia's treatment team.

with the psychiatrist. Andy's case manager sees him at school once a week to help him get along better with peers. She also does an activity with Andy after school, which has the added benefit of providing some respite for Connie. The probation officer works with Andy on taking responsibility for his actions and is available for Connie to call on during crises.

• *Use your resources well.* If you know the scope and goals of each service, you can more effectively evaluate their usefulness and use them to their fullest. Your psychiatrist will be most effective if you provide meaningful information about symptoms and side effects (see Chapter 4 for ideas about keeping records). Your therapy will be most helpful if you make a good effort to try suggestions and if you follow through on assignments between sessions. Therapy will also be more effective if you provide honest feedback about suggestions.

• *Communication between providers.* You can facilitate communication between providers by choosing providers who can easily confer on a regular basis. For example, some psychiatrists work in clinics with psychologists and social workers on staff. In this type of setting, it's easy for your providers to stay in close contact because they work together on a daily basis. Every time you have a session, your providers will make notes about the session in your chart. When your providers work in the same setting, they will share the chart and therefore see each other's notes. If you can't find providers who work in the same clinic, you can ask the person with whom you initiate treatment (i.e., the person who does your evaluation) to suggest other providers with whom he has a good working relationship (e.g., ask your psychologist for the name of a psychiatrist).

Having multiple treatment providers, all with different roles, can result in optimal care and maximum benefit for your child. When treatment goes well, you work with each provider on a different set of goals, and the various providers communicate effectively with you and with each other.

However, even with the best of intentions, having multiple providers can sometimes be difficult. You may get confusing, contradictory messages—a sign that you need to reexamine your mental health team and determine whether all providers are truly helpful and/or whether better communication is necessary. There is also a significant practical problem with having a number of providers: seeing and paying for all the providers can drain the family of precious resources—both time and money. Your goal is to get as much assistance as you need, but not too much.

Your child is unlikely to need all of the interventions described in this chapter. However, as your child's case manager, it's important that you understand how to assemble an effective treatment team. You choose providers, schedule appointments, and ultimately evaluate the effectiveness of the services you receive. You also administer medications, follow through on recommendations, and support your child on a day-to-day basis. So continue reading. In Chapters 6 and 7 we delve further into the different treatments for mood disorders. Reading those chapters will help equip you to build and evaluate your mental health team.

6 | What Do Medications Offer?

Many of the parents we've known have approached the subject of medication for their child's mood disorder with trepidation: Are psychotropic drugs safe for children, especially young ones? Will medication become a crutch that the child will never be able to cast off? Will the side effects be as difficult for the child to handle as the mood symptoms have been? Will evening out the child's moods turn him or her into a different person? In this chapter we answer questions such as these and help you weigh the pros and cons so you can decide whether medication will be of overall benefit to your child.

First, understand that medications do not *cure* mood disorders. They are, however, an important part of *managing* depressive and bipolar illnesses. Medication can:

- *Stop* or *lessen* current symptom severity
- *Prevent* or *decrease* impairment from future episodes.

Medications *do not* solve every problem that mood disorders bring. As discussed in Chapter 4, some co-occurring symptoms go away with medications, whereas others require therapy (see Chapter 7). Some symptoms improve with medication but do not go away. For medications to do their best, it's essential that you function as an *active partner* in treatment.

Becoming an Active Partner

Being an active partner requires your involvement from the treatment-planning stages through the course of your child's illness. As we've said, the first step is conducting a meaningful and realistic cost–benefit analysis.

To Medicate or Not to Medicate: The Cost–Benefit Analysis

Ten-year-old Mike was recently diagnosed with bipolar disorder Type II, and his parents were agonizing over whether to approve treating their son with medication. Wouldn't the mood stabilizer that the doctor was suggesting diminish Mike's creativity, change his personality in ways that no one would want? Mike had always been viewed as the "life of the party" and was well liked by both teachers and peers. But his typically upbeat mood in social settings could give way to irritability and desperate sadness at home, at least for short periods, and his very high energy level and need to move rapidly from one highly stimulating activity to another was draining for his family and a strain on his teachers. It was mainly Mike's aggressiveness toward his younger sister during periods of irritability, though, that had made his parents consider medication.

Mike's treatment began with a combination of individual and family therapy with a therapist well versed in childhood mood disorders. With the help of their therapist, Mike and his family became increasingly aware of Mike's target symptoms—moods that changed rapidly from elated to angry to sad, racing thoughts, high activity level—and the impact of those symptoms on Mike and those around him. While Mike's therapist worked with Mike and his parents to develop ways to tame Mike's wild mood swings, she also introduced the idea of a medication evaluation by a child and adolescent psychiatrist. Mike's parents were hesitant about putting Mike on medication, fearful of side effects, of the stigma associated with being on medication for behavior change, and of the long-term consequences of "drugging" their child. After several months of thinking about the issue and participating in therapy, however, Mike and his parents decided to meet with the psychiatrist. The psychiatrist recommended a trial on a mood stabilizer and also encouraged Mike and his family to continue working with their therapist on the many issues that arise for families of children with bipolar disorder. In therapy, Mike's family addressed sibling concerns and developed an effective school coping plan, which was shared with Mike's teacher and principal. Also, Mike and his parents had a reliable place to vent, to express their fears, frustrations, and worries, and to develop plans with an experienced "navigator" to manage the very symptoms that had generated those negative feelings.

After he started on lithium, Mike's mood became more stable, with fewer and less extreme ups and downs. As a result, his relationships with family members improved. Mike did experience some tremor that interfered with his schoolwork and drawing. This effect was reduced by altering the amount and timing of his doses. He also dreaded the blood draws and spent a therapy session developing ways to reduce his aversion to the process. Mike continued to be creative, and as his energy level returned to normal, it became easier for peers to relate to him, and his friendships grew.

Mike's family provides us with a great example of a careful cost–benefit analysis. They sought an evaluation when his symptoms began to create stress at home, used therapy to learn about Mike's diagnosis and to develop coping skills, and then made a careful decision about initiating medications. Although medications could not do everything for Mike, they were helpful.

Organizing and Maintaining Your Child's Records

You are the eyes and ears of your child's treatment team. Except when home-based interventions are provided (and even then, the home-based therapist isn't there all the time), your treatment providers are unlikely to see your child at home. You're the one who sees the rages, the chronic irritability, or the despairing tears. In fact, many children seem to have a knack for pulling themselves together in time for therapy sessions. This is the reason your recorded observations become important. When your daughter is having a rage precipitated by your serving hamburgers for dinner, the situation is vivid to you. However, by the time of your appointment with the psychiatrist next week, your memory will have faded somewhat. So you will be well served by maintaining useful records about your child. We recommend that you start with a large loose-leaf binder containing several section dividers, as you will be most organized if you keep different types of records in each of the sections. We've outlined some "rules" to follow in developing and maintaining your child's binder.

1. *Keep a record of mood symptoms.* We've provided three examples of mood charts in Chapter 4. Rating mood symptoms numerically simplifies the information and allows you to see progress or decline graphically. It's particularly important to track mood symptoms during medication trials. This information will guide medication decisions.

2. *Write down events when they happen.* Keep some blank paper in your binder. When something unusual occurs, take some notes. If the event is serious, you might need to call your doctor to report it. Having notes in front of you when you speak to your doctor may help you describe what occurred. If the situation is not an emergency, having the notes will assist you in sharing the information at your next appointment.

Remember Andy? He's the eleven-year-old with rapid-cycling bipolar disorder from Chapter 5. One month into treatment, Andy started acting strangely. He began holding his ears and shaking his head violently. At first he ran away and lashed out at his mother when she tried to hold him. Once Connie was able to hold him, Andy screamed and cried for twenty minutes, then fell asleep in her arms. Once he was settled, Connie jotted down a few notes and called his psychiatrist. The psychiatrist called her back two hours later, and she was able to give him a detailed description of what had happened. The psychiatrist instructed her to take Andy to the emergency room if he became too violent or agitated to manage at home and to be sure to keep Andy's scheduled appointment with his therapist the next day. When Andy saw his therapist the next day, she determined that Andy was hearing voices. She provided that information to the psychiatrist, who prescribed an antipsychotic medication for Andy.

3. *Keep a medication log.* It's important to maintain a careful record of the medications your child takes (and has taken). This record should include your child's weight at the time a new medicine is prescribed (or when the dose of an existing medicine is changed), how he or she responded to the medicine, and what, if any, side effects he or she has experienced. From our personal experience, it's incredibly helpful when we conduct evaluations if parents can tell us exactly what has and has not worked for their child. This aids the diagnostic process and certainly guides future treatment. Having a comprehensive treatment log is also exceedingly helpful if you change prescribing physicians—which is

not an infrequent occurrence, because specialists move, insurance coverage changes, people relocate for jobs or other needs, or you may need to find a more compatible fit with a new provider. We suggest you take your binder to appointments; that will allow you to take notes and to incorporate any new papers you get during sessions.

4. *Always ask for fact sheets (from your physician or pharmacy) about medications and save them in your binder.* These sheets typically have information about side effects. They provide a convenient reference if your child ever experiences a side effect and you aren't sure how serious it is (of course, you should always call your prescribing physician if a side effect seems serious).

5. *Write questions in your binder when they occur to you.* Getting into the habit of always taking your binder with you to appointments will help you remember to ask all these questions. Also, jotting down your treatment provider's answer at the appointment will decrease the likelihood that you'll need to cover the same ground repeatedly. You have too much to remember on a daily basis—don't rely on your memory for important questions or their answers.

6. *Share the information—all of it. Always* tell both your primary care doctor and your psychiatrist about *all* medications (including over-the-counter remedies, herbal treatments, and nutritional supplements) your child is taking. *Many mood disorder medications can interact with other medications, remedies, and dietary supplements.* We recommend that you fill all your child's prescriptions at the same pharmacy. That way the pharmacist will also be aware if you are doubling up on medicines that should not be taken together.

Learning to Monitor Your Child's Treatment

You're the person who is with your child most and knows your child best, so your treatment team will rely on your help to monitor your child's progress. When a new medication is prescribed, be sure to learn about its potential side effects. Medications may have relatively common mild, or "nuisance," side effects and, less commonly, some serious side effects. You need to know which side effects are serious, how to recognize them, and what to do if you notice them—both during regular business hours and after hours. You need to know what number to call during your prescribing physician's regular office hours and after hours, as well as where to turn (e.g., a hospital emergency room or an urgent care facility) if your child needs to be evaluated face to face.

WEIGHING THE COST OF SIDE EFFECTS

Although many aspects of Mike's life improved significantly with medication, he had to learn to cope with some annoying side effects. After about a month of taking his medication regularly, he noticed that his pants were getting tight. His mother had mentioned that he seemed to be eating more than usual and that it seemed he was always hungry. To combat the problem, Mike started trying to choose more fruits and vegetables for snacks and added walking the family dog to his routine every afternoon. Side effects such as minor weight gain may be simply a nuisance and can be countered using simple measures, but others may require you to change your child's medications (or, in some cases, add another medication). You may decide to accept some mild side effects if the medication is effective in improving your child's overall level of functioning. For example, you may be willing to accept a slight tremor if, after your child has tried many medications previously, the current medications are allowing him to function at school and to begin to make friends for the first time. Depending on your child, there also may be side effects you are unwilling to accept, such as significant weight gain or bed-wetting in an older child.

REMEMBER THE "OBSERVER EFFECT"

When Mike and his family initially made the decision for Mike to start medication, he was very wary. His psychiatrist gave him a list of the possible side effects. For the first couple of weeks he was sure he was experiencing every one of them. Over time he became accustomed to the medication and learned to cope with only the few minor side effects that he did experience. Just as some medical students start to wonder if they have the diseases they're studying, or pregnant women may start paying attention to every physical twinge they experience, it's easy to credit new medicines with more side effects than they actually produce. Although parents should always be aware of side effects that might occur, they should also be aware of the "observer effect." This refers to the common experience of noticing many little things that have always been there once you start to monitor possible side effects. For example, one possible side effect of a new medicine may be an upset stomach. If your child has had frequent stomachaches as part of his depression, experiencing them after beginning the new medicine may continue to reflect his depression, not the treatment for it.

MONITORING TREATMENT RESPONSE

In addition to monitoring side effects, it's important to monitor your child's treatment response. You can use one of the mood logs we presented in Chapter 4 or just jot down observations in your child's treatment binder if this fits better with your family's pace. It's very useful to understand which "target symptoms" are expected to be affected by each medication your child takes. For example, a child might be prescribed Depakote (an anticonvulsant that works as a mood stabilizer) to reduce rages, grandiosity, and racing thoughts; Zoloft (an antidepressant) to reduce anxiety; and Adderall (a stimulant) to increase concentration and reduce impulsivity. If you know what each medication is supposed to do, you'll be able to evaluate its effectiveness more accurately.

Ensuring Treatment Adherence

At first it may seem pretty easy to remember to give your child his medication or to remind an older child to take it on time. After all, this is a new element in your lives, and you're pretty tuned in to it. But as time goes on, it's easy to get lax, and missed medication can compromise all the gains your child has made through treatment. So have a plan (and a backup plan) for making sure medication is taken as prescribed. We are firm believers in the use of a pill holder labeled with the days of the week in which you place your child's pills once a week. This plan not only helps you monitor the daily ritual of pill taking but also helps you remember to get refills on time. We also suggest that you develop little rituals around pill taking (e.g., your child always gets a glass of his favorite juice to wash the pills down) and that you keep medications in a place that will easily remind you to have your child take them.

No matter how organized you are, however, sooner or later you'll probably miss a dose of medication, and it's important to know ahead of time what to do about it. This is one of those questions to write down in your binder to ask your prescribing physician at a regular appointment: Should your child take the missed dose as soon as you remember, or should you skip this dose and just take the next one? Or does it depend on how much time has elapsed? Whatever the doctor's instructions, be sure to keep a record of missed doses and to be honest with your treatment team about missed medication. If in reality your child is taking only 50 percent of his medication and you report continuing symptoms without reporting missed doses, your treatment team is likely to think the medications aren't working and suggest an unnecessary change in medication or dosage.

WHO'S IN CHARGE?

A question we frequently deal with in therapy sessions is, "Who is supposed to be in charge of remembering the medicine?" Our answer differs, based on the child's age and other family factors. With elementary school children, we recommend that parents assume full responsibility for remembering and administering medication. For "tweens" (eleven- to thirteen-year-olds or middle-schoolers), we work with families to make a transition plan—one in which the child begins to take on increasing responsibility. Using a pill box makes this transition plan easier. If your daughter knows where her pill box is, she can take her morning medicine with her juice before you come downstairs in the morning, or your son can take his evening pill between his favorite TV shows. You are available as the backup to remind your child if she hasn't already taken care of the job. The goal is for adolescents (high school students) to be even more responsible for taking their medication. Again, we suggest that Mom or Dad be a reliable backup prompter. Be aware that most schools will not allow your child to have medications with him during the school day. If doses are not taken at home, be sure that the school nurse or another school official is informed and that the medications are stored with that person and that the appropriate forms are signed.

YET ANOTHER BATTLEGROUND?

With any age child, if battles occur over taking the medicine, it's time for your family to talk. We suggest you hold a parent–child meeting to clarify the pros and cons of taking medication and to develop a revised plan for how that will be accomplished. (In Chapter 8 we discuss in more detail how to improve communication and problem solving with regard to symptom management. A very common application of these newly improved skills is to develop medication plans that are acceptable to all family members.)

If you still feel stuck after holding a family meeting, bring this issue up at your next appointment with your prescribing physician and/or therapist. Your treatment provider may have suggestions your family hasn't tried yet or may be able to help your child work through his concerns about the medicine. Some common reasons children don't like taking a particular medication include the shape, size, or taste of the pill. Sometimes adjustments can be made by switching to a different form of the medication, by crushing the medicine (although not all medicines can be handled this way) and putting it in applesauce, or by taking the medication with another food (e.g., pudding) or drink (e.g., chocolate milk) that will hide the flavor.

For older children and teenagers, resistance to taking medications may be caused by not wanting to feel different from their friends, not wanting others to know they're taking medication (especially at overnight gatherings), concern that medications are addictive or that taking medications is like taking street drugs, or dislike of the medication's side effects. These are all issues your child or teen may work through, in a discussion with you and/or with the assistance of her therapist. Respecting your child's opinion and feelings, while providing information relevant to the discussion at hand (e.g., many teenagers take medicine, they just might not talk about it; psychotropic medicines aren't addictive; these medicines work to bring your brain back to baseline, not to alter it the way street drugs do), working out arrangements more suitable to your teen (e.g., providing a small pill holder so your child can take her medicine privately while at a sleepover), and working proactively with the prescribing physician to minimize side effects (e.g., changing when the medicine is taken, dividing one dose into two, or taking medicine with food) are all important steps, and convey to your adolescent that you respect his concerns and are willing to work together to address his issues.

Managing Side Effects

Although your prescribing physician will try to keep side effects to a minimum, sometimes side effects have to be accepted to get the benefit of medication. Learning strategies to minimize the impact of side effects can reduce resistance to taking medications and improve quality of life for your child and you. The sidebar presents a series of tips that have helped many children deal with unwanted side effects. First, though, we've summarized several larger principles about medication usage common to any medicine your child might require.

Many side effects decrease as the body adjusts to the medicine. So, if side effects emerge shortly after your child starts a new medication, don't despair. These side effects might go away with time. Sometimes changing the amount or timing of doses can help reduce unwanted side effects. Alternatively, switching to a slightly different medication can be helpful. *Remember our motto: It's not your fault but it is your challenge!* So share your observations with your treatment providers, ask questions, and seek new and helpful information. Encourage your child to become an active participant in her treatment as well.

It All Takes Time

Initially, a new medicine may work only partially, so you might notice 50 percent improvement. When that happens, the glass is both half full and half empty. You're on the road to recovery, but you haven't gotten there yet. Hang in there, and keep working with your treatment team. Partial responses are common. Sometimes a change in dose is needed. Some medications have to be increased slowly over time, and some need to reach a particular concentration in the system before they become effective. These gradual dose increases may take a while. Be patient—if you push your prescribing physician into making a change too quickly, you'll never know how effective the first medicine could have been. Having a trusting relationship with a competent prescribing physician becomes particularly important in these cases. You need to be able to trust your physician to change or increase doses in a safe and effective manner. In some cases, simply changing the timing of doses can improve functioning considerably.

TIPS FOR PARENTS: MANAGING COMMON SIDE EFFECTS

Dizziness: Stand up slowly.

Dry mouth: Drink water, chew sugarless gum or candy.

Constipation: Eat high-fiber diet (whole grains, fruit, and raw vegetables). Drink plenty of water (it fills you up with no added calories or artificial sweeteners).

Upset stomach/nausea: Take medication with food or in divided doses.

Increased thirst: Drink water (arrange access at school), avoid caffeine.

Increased urination: Arrange bathroom breaks.

Weight gain: Increase exercise, eat low-fat diet, drink plenty of water (not high-calorie juice or soda), eat lots of fiber to help fill you up, avoid junk food.

Tremor: Take medication with meals or in divided doses, avoid caffeine.

Skin sensitivity: Use sunscreen, wear protective clothing, avoid sunlight and sunlamps.

Impaired sleep: Keep a consistent sleep routine, don't let the weekend disrupt sleep routines by more than one hour, no exercise or caffeine in the evening, wake at a regular time (even if tired), don't nap during the day!

After the addition of therapy, case management, placement in a specialized classroom, and dietary supplementation, Andy (age eleven) was functioning better but continued to have very difficult evenings. During the month between appointments with Andy's psychiatrist, Connie kept careful records and got feedback from his teachers. Andy was doing better at school but seemed sleepy in the morning. Meanwhile, his moods fluctuated considerably in the evening, and Andy was having significant trouble settling down to go to sleep. When Connie mentioned this, Andy's psychiatrist suggested keeping his total amount of medication the same but giving him half of his Risperdal in the morning and half in the early evening instead of the whole dose in the morning.

By dividing his dose, they eliminated an unwanted side effect, and symptom management was improved without increasing Andy's medication. Connie's careful records, which included documentation of her communication with Andy's teacher, provided the psychiatrist with the information she needed to be able to make this helpful adjustment.

For some children the type of medication needs to be changed. Anya, age eleven, has a long history of behavioral problems and clear symptoms of bipolar disorder. After finally being evaluated by a child and adolescent psychiatrist well versed in early-onset mood disorders, Anya was prescribed a mood stabilizer. Much to her parents' disappointment, Anya showed significant side effects but not much improvement. She was then switched to a different mood stabilizer, again with little success. At that point the psychiatrist recommended changing from mood stabilizers to an atypical antipsychotic, a class of medications that can be very helpful in stabilizing the moods of children with bipolar disorder, particularly those who do not respond well to traditional mood stabilizers. This new medication was helpful for Anya, and for the first time in a long time her mother began to feel hopeful.

SETTING REALISTIC EXPECTATIONS

Many medicines take several weeks or more to work. If you don't know this about a new prescription, you might be sorely disappointed when your child doesn't begin to show a positive response within forty-eight hours, so be sure to ask. Jarrod is eight and cycles daily between extreme anger, out-of-control elation, and desperate sadness. During rages, he is destructive and aggressive toward his parents, and at other times he is giddy, silly, and seems to "bounce off the walls." He was seen by a psychiatrist who was a provider for the family's insurance plan. Jarrod was initially started on a mood stabilizer. After a one-month trial on the same dose with no response, Jarrod was switched to a different mood stabilizer. At the next visit two weeks later, his medication was changed again.

Jarrod's father, Rob, became concerned that the psychiatrist did not seem to have a good understanding of his son's needs and began doing some research on the Internet. Rob decided that they needed to see a specialist in child and adolescent mood disorders. He spoke with the benefits coordinator at his office, who helped him convince the insurance company to cover a child and adolescent psychiatrist in the neighboring community. Due to the previous rapid changes between medications, their new doctor suggested starting all over again with longer trials on each medication. After several months that included gradual dose increases, Jarrod improved significantly on the initial medication.

If you give up on a medication too soon and switch, you'll never know whether that medication would have been effective—a hazard that arises mainly when the prescriber is unfamiliar with childhood mood disorders, as in Jarrod's case. At the same time, sticking with an ineffective medication or dose for an excessive amount of time is not helpful, either. Ten-year old Krystal was seen by her family doctor for increasing sadness, withdrawal from her friends and family, trouble falling asleep at night, loss of appetite, and difficulty staying focused on her schoolwork. The doctor agreed to start her on an antidepressant as long as Krystal also saw a therapist. He told Krystal's mother, Janette, to call or come back if she had any problems and that he wanted to see Krystal in two months. Janette was very hopeful and kept watching Krystal for signs of improvement. Three months went by. Janette hadn't made an appointment for therapy yet, so she kept delaying making a follow-up appointment with Dr. Carson. Finally, the doctor's office called Janette because Dr. Carson was concerned that he hadn't seen Krystal. After learning she had not improved, he increased the dose. Ten days after the dose increase, Janette began to notice significant improvements. First, Krystal began to fall asleep more easily and to eat healthy meals again. Next, Janette noticed that Krystal's mood was more cheerful and her attitude was more positive. Meanwhile, Janette finally made an appointment with a social worker, who helped Krystal get back on track with her schoolwork and friends.

Krystal's response to medication followed a common pattern that you should be alert for. Her physical symptoms (sleep and appetite changes) improved before her mood and thinking began to change.

WHY DOES MY CHILD'S BLOOD NEED TO BE TESTED?

1. To enhance effectiveness. The same dose of medicine can produce different blood concentration levels in different people. Some medications have a known range of therapeutic concentration levels. Tracking levels of medicine in the blood can help guide dose increases or decreases to achieve a level in the therapeutic range.
2. To monitor safety. Medications are processed by different organs. When a medication is processed primarily by the kidneys or the liver, the functioning of these organs can be monitored to ensure that the medication is being tolerated well by the body.

How Are Levels Taken?

1. Your child's doctor will give you a written order for a blood test.
2. On the designated day, you'll go to the laboratory of your choice (some are better equipped to work with children than others).
3. Blood levels should be taken twelve hours after the last dose of medication (first thing in the morning is usually best).
4. The level should be taken *before the next dose,* which means that the morning dose should be postponed until after the blood is drawn.
5. If your child has significant and ongoing difficulty with necessary blood draws, and if providing incentives and practice has not helped, talk to your doctor. Creams are available that numb the skin prior to a blood test (e.g., Emla Cream). These creams typically have to be applied in advance of the blood draw (i.e., one hour) and can be expensive.

WHAT IF THINGS GO WELL?

Achieving a full response to the medication (i.e., eliminating symptoms altogether) is *not* a reason to discontinue medication. Once symptoms of the most recent episode are controlled, the goal of using medication switches to preventing future episodes. As we discussed in Chapter 3, recent research has shown that mood episodes tend to increase in frequency and severity over time, so prevention of future episodes is critical. If after careful consideration you decide to discontinue some or all medications or to reduce them to a maintenance dose, develop a plan with your doctor concerning both when and how to stop or reduce the medicine. If and when you decide to stop a medication, input from your doctor can spare you some unpleasant surprises. Stopping abruptly may lead to nasty and unnecessary side effects, so a careful plan to taper medications may be needed.

WHAT IF THINGS STOP GOING WELL?

Remember, your child is developing physically. This means his body is a moving target, and dose adjustments will be needed over time. Even keeping this in mind, however, we frequently hear another complaint from parents. Medicine that has been working for a long time suddenly stops working—and no other obvious changes (such as moving from middle school to high school or your teenager's best friend's moving away) have occurred. Although we don't have a good explanation for this in the scientific literature, it is something we see fairly regularly. If this happens to your child, get right back in to see your psychiatrist. You may need to switch to another medication to "freshen up" the treatment response.

A Primer on Medications

Entire books have been written about psychiatric medications for children (see the Resources for further reading). We suggest you review those books to learn more about the medications your child has been prescribed. Also, your prescribing physician and pharmacist should have fact sheets about any medicine your child takes. It is important to keep these available for reference, as many medications can interact with other prescribed medications, over-the-counter remedies, and herbal products.

Our goal here is to give you some basic information about "classes," or types, of medicines to provide you with a common language to use with your treatment providers. Keep in mind that none of the medications discussed in this section are addictive. This is a common misconception that leads some people to delay getting needed treatment.

Classes of Medications

Although medications are often named based on the disorders they are most frequently used to treat, these names sometimes can be misleading. For example, some antidepressants are used (very effectively) to reduce anxiety. Keep in mind that medications are used to treat particular symptoms or sets of symptoms, not disorders.

Some classes of medications contain subgroups. These subgroups are usually based on *how* medications work and which neurotransmitters (chemicals responsible for communication in the brain) they target.

A note to weary parents: Research is ongoing. As you are reading, the search continues for new, more effective medications with fewer side effects. So stay hopeful and keep trying.

Antidepressants

It is important to note that if a child with bipolar disorder takes an antidepressant *without* already being prescribed a mood stabilizer (described later), he may become manic or hypomanic. There may also be the risk of activation if the child is on a mood stabilizer. Recent studies of depressed children have also shown activation on several antidepressants (e.g., Paxil and Effexor). For these reasons, it is very important to have a careful diagnosis (including questions about family history and a wide array of possible symptoms) before launching any medication treatment, and to monitor treatment response closely afterward.

SSRIS

The most commonly prescribed subgroup of antidepressants is the SSRIs (selective serotonin reuptake inhibitors). These medications increase the amount of serotonin in the brain and thereby reduce depressive symptoms. The SSRIs are typically considered "first line" (meaning they are tried first) medications for depression, as well as for some anxiety disorders, including obsessive–compulsive disorder, generalized anxiety disorder, and social phobia. Table 2 provides a list of the SSRIs with both their generic and brand names. Although all the SSRIs in-

TABLE 2 Generic and Brand Names of SSRI Antidepressants	
Generic name	Brand name
fluoxetine	Prozac
sertraline	Zoloft
fluvoxamine	Luvox
paroxetine	Paxil
citalopram	Celexa
escitalopram	Lexapro

crease availability of serotonin in the brain, they vary in their chemical structures, the rate at which they are broken down in the body, and their side effects. SSRIs tend to have mild side effects with less sedation, cardiovascular, and weight-gain side effects than some of the older antidepressants.

Common side effects of SSRI may include dizziness, nausea, stomachaches, diarrhea, nervousness or agitation, drowsiness or insomnia, increase or decrease in appetite, weakness, dry mouth, tremor, and increased perspiration. We refer to these as mild side effects—they may cause significant discomfort and need management strategies, but they are not life threatening. Possible serious side effects of SSRIs include triggering mania, seizures, or suicidality. If you ever suspect a serious side effect, contact your physician. Above all else, never ignore your gut instinct—it's a powerful parental tool!

ATYPICAL ANTIDEPRESSANTS

The atypical antidepressants include several medications that differ from each other and from the SSRIs in a variety of ways.

Wellbutrin (generic name, *bupropion*) is a unique antidepressant with a chemical structure similar to that of some of the stimulants. It's particularly useful for depressed children with co-occurring ADHD, especially those unable to tolerate stimulant medications. Wellbutrin is less likely than other antidepressants to cause behavioral activation (e.g., hypomania or mania) and therefore is useful for children with significant mood swings, a history of activation on other antidepressants, or a family history of bipolar disorder. Wellbutrin is also approved under the name Zyban as a smoking cessation aid. Side effects include irritability, decreased appetite, insomnia, and worsening of tics. Irritability may be a signal that the dose needs to be lowered. Wellbutrin also carries a higher risk of medication-induced seizures, which is particularly relevant for children with a history of seizures and for individuals who binge and purge (i.e., children or adolescents with bulimia or symptoms of bulimia).

Effexor (venlafaxine) is similar to the SSRIs in that it increases serotonin but also increases another neurotransmitter called *norepinephrine,* or *noradrenaline*. Side effects may include nausea, agitation, stomachaches, headaches, increased blood pressure, and increased suicidality.

Serzone (nefazodone) and *Desyrel (trazodone)* are similar to each other and are useful for depression, anxiety, and sleep problems. One of their most significant side effects is sedation, which can be a helpful side effect for a child or adolescent who is having difficulty sleeping. Other side effects include agitation, dry mouth, and constipation.

Also sedating, *Remeron (mirtazapine)* can be useful for children or adolescents who have difficulty sleeping. Other side effects include "heaviness" and upset stomach.

TRICYCLIC ANTIDEPRESSANTS (TCAS) AND MONOAMINE OXIDASE INHIBITORS (MAOIS)

Currently, tricyclic antidepressants (TCAs) are used more for ADHD (as third-line choices) and tic disorders than for childhood depression. Examples of tricyclics include Elavil (amitriptyline), Pamelor (nortriptyline), Tofranil (imipramine), and Anafranil (clomipramine).

The monoamine oxidase inhibitors (*MAOIs*) are the oldest class of antidepressants and are very effective. Unfortunately, they require strict dietary limitations (no aged foods and no aged cheeses) and are almost never used for childhood depression. Examples include Parnate and Nardil.

Herbal Remedies

Herbal remedies, although not controlled by the Food and Drug Administration (FDA), are medications. A number of herbal remedies (e.g., wild oats, lemon balm, ginseng, wood betony, basil, rhodiola rosea) have been suggested as being beneficial for depression. Only St. John's wort (*Hypericum perforatum*) has been demonstrated as effective through controlled research. Klaus Linde and his colleagues at Munich University found that St. John's wort worked as well as standard antidepressants in adults with mild and moderate depression. Because St. John's wort has a lower rate of side effects, it has been suggested as a safe and effective alternative for mild and moderate depression. Bob Findling and colleagues in Cleveland have found St. John's wort safe and beneficial in a small study of children aged 6–16. They recommend further study of it. Possible side effects of St. John's wort include upset stomach, dry mouth, fatigue, dizziness, rashes, and itching. St. John's wort can also cause birth control pills to lose their effectiveness.

SAM-e has also been investigated as an herbal remedy for depression. It also has not been studied in children. The only documented side effect of SAM-e is upset stomach.

Melatonin is another herbal remedy that can be helpful for individuals with mood disorders. Melatonin can be useful as a sleep aid. Its possible side effects include feeling sedated in the mornings and changes in dream activity.

Keep in mind that herbal remedies are not regulated by the FDA. This means that there is no guarantee that the concentration of the active ingredient is consistent between brands and even between batches. It can be difficult to choose a brand and determine how much to take.

Mood Stabilizers

Mood stabilizers are used to reduce manic symptoms and to control mood cycling. The first mood stabilizer to be discovered was lithium, and it continues to be effective and commonly used.

Tegretol (carbamazepine) and Depakote (valproic acid; other brand names include Valproate and Depakene) are anticonvulsants used to treat epilepsy. They work by reducing abnormal brain activity in the parts of the brain that control emotions and thus are good mood stabilizers. They are used in bipolar disorder to control mania and reduce mood cycling. There is debate over Depakote's possible linkage with polycystic ovary disorder in females. If your daughter is prescribed Depa-

---

MEDICATION INFORMATION: LITHIUM (ESKALITH, ESKALITH CR, LITHANE, LITHOBID, LITHONATE, AND LITHOTABS)

1. Lithium must be monitored with blood draws.
   a. To establish blood levels (to verify that levels are in the therapeutic range)
   b. Periodic tests of kidney functioning needed as it is excreted by the kidney
   c. Thyroid levels should be monitored throughout treatment

2. Lithium is a salt.
   a. Avoid salt-restricted diets
   b. Maintain regular liquid intake and don't limit fluids (get extra fluids if you exercise or get hot)

3. Common side effects include nausea, cramps, fatigue, slight weakness, or dizziness—these may subside; thirstiness, increased urination, bed-wetting, tremor, weight gain, acne worsening

4. Serious side effects caused by lithium toxicity include slurred speech, confusion, impaired walking, vomiting, diarrhea, severe tremors, muscle twitching, blurred vision, irregular pulse. *If these occur, contact your doctor—your child's lithium level may be too high!*

5. Avoid ibuprofen (Advil, Motrin, Nuprin, Midol)

**MEDICATION INFORMATION:
DEPAKOTE (VALPROIC ACID,
DEPAKENE, VALPROATE)**

---

1. Must be monitored with blood draws.
   a. To check levels of medication in the blood (to verify that levels are in the therapeutic range).
   b. Liver functioning should be checked (prior to starting and every six months thereafter) as it is processed and excreted by the liver.

2. Common side effects include nausea, vomiting, indigestion, drowsiness, and weight gain.

3. Serious side effects include weakness, facial swelling, loss of energy, weight loss. *If these occur, contact your doctor!*

4. Avoid aspirin

5. Life-threatening pancreatitis has occurred in a very small number of persons taking Depakote. Severe abdominal pain should be immediately reported to your doctor.

kote, talk with your prescribing physician about this concern.

NEW MOOD-STABILIZING
ANTICONVULSANTS

We mention these because they are potentially promising treatments for bipolar disorder, but the research is very limited, especially in children. See Table 3 for the names and side effects of these medications.

Atypical Antipsychotics

The atypical antipsychotics are an increasingly important tool in treating childhood mood disorders, especially bipolar disorder. In addition to controlling psychotic symptoms (hallucinations, delusions), they decrease agitation and aggression. Importantly, their mood-stabilizing effects have been observed clinically and are being demonstrated through research. The

| TABLE 3 | New Mood Stabilizers |

Brand name	Side effects
Topamax	Fatigue, dizziness, nervousness, tingling arms and/or legs
Gabitril	Fatigue, dizziness, unstable gait
Lamictal	Not advised for children—used for adolescents Skin rash (can be serious, more common in children), blurred or double vision, fatigue, dizziness
Trileptal	Weight loss, rash, sedation

atypical antipsychotics are also used on a short-term basis when psychotic symptoms occur along with depression. These medications include Risperdal (risperidone), Seroquel (quetiapine), Zyprexa (olanzapine), Clozaril (clozapine), Abilify (aripiprazole), and Geodon (ziprasidone). Common side effects include drowsiness, increased appetite, weight gain, slowing, tremor, tenseness, and a "masked" face. An infrequent but serious set of side effects includes severe muscle tightness, confusion, sweating, fever, and unstable blood pressure and pulse. In the case of side effects resembling this list, contact your physician immediately or go to the emergency room.

**MEDICATION INFORMATION:
TEGRETOL (CARBAMAZEPINE)**

1. Must be monitored with blood draws.
   a. To check levels of medication in the blood.
   b. Liver functioning should be checked (prior to starting, after six weeks, and every six months after that) as it is processed and excreted by the liver.
   c. Can reduce white blood cell count; check blood counts periodically if a serious sore throat or infection occurs.

2. Dose is often increased in two to six weeks.

3. Common side effects include drowsiness, clumsiness, dizziness, nausea/vomiting.

4. Less common side effects include muscle or joint aches, constipation or diarrhea, dry mouth, headache, increased sensitivity to sunlight, sore throat, hair loss, increased perspiring, sexual problems, unusual bleeding or bruising.

5. May interact with antibiotics, cough and cold remedies, and birth control pills, resulting in either decreased effectiveness or serious side effects.

6. *Call your doctor about sore throats or fever!*

Antihypertensives

Clonidine and Tenex are commonly prescribed medications for lowering blood pressure. In children with mood disorders, they're used to decrease agitation, to assist with sleep, and to reduce impulsivity and tics. Their most common side effects are drowsiness (they are often prescribed specifically for this side effect) and dizziness.

Common Manic Triggers

We mentioned previously that antidepressants (including herbal remedies) can trigger mania or hypomania in children who have bipolar disorder and who are not already on mood stabilizers. For that reason, children with bipolar disorder typically do best if the medication prescribed for their manic symptoms is working well to stabilize mood before either an antidepressant or a stimulant is started. If you recall, Amy in Chapter 5 had her "piles" of problems treated in precisely that order.

There are several other manic triggers that parents of children with bipolar disorder (or parents of children with depression, if there is a family history of bipolar disorder) should be aware of, as these may also ignite manic or hypomanic symptoms in their child.

MANIC TRIGGERS

Steroid medications (if needed for asthma control, work carefully with both prescribing physicians—make sure they each know all the medications your child is taking)

Pseudoephedrine (found in Sudafed and some other over-the-counter cough/cold remedies)

Caffeine (in particular, dysregulated sleep can lead to mania)

Drugs of abuse (e.g., cocaine, Ecstasy)

The decision to start medications for your child can be a complicated one. You will need to weigh the cost of the mood symptoms (e.g., disrupted social relationships, failure to progress in school, not enjoying life) against the potential side effects of medications. Mood disorders can wreak havoc on development—so much is changing in the life of a child and so much important growth needs to occur. Be sure to make an informed decision about medications with the support and advice of professionals you trust.

Finally, it's very important to remember that medications are an integral component of managing mood disorders but should not be the *sole* treatment. Other nonpharmacological interventions, discussed in greater detail in Chapters 5 and 7 through 10, can also change your child's physical and emotional status. Remember that good sleep hygiene, regular exercise, enjoyable activities, and a healthy diet are "free" medicines. They are an important part of good self-care, they help to control stress, and they can reduce some mood symptoms. On the flip side, not keeping a regular sleep routine, being inactive, and eating too much junk food can compound your child's problems.

7 | What Should I Expect from Therapy?

Medications are an important *part* of the package of interventions for mood disorders. Many illnesses may be treated with medication but, for best results, should be treated with behavioral, emotional, and environmental changes as well. Diabetes, for example, is treated with insulin, but people with diabetes must also monitor their diets, exercise regularly, and manage stress effectively. Taking insulin alone results in only partial control of the illness. Like diabetes, mood disorders are biological illnesses that are largely influenced by psychological and environmental factors.

Therapy for children and adolescents with mood disorders can help with symptom management, relapse prevention, maximizing functioning, managing co-occurring disorders, and improving peer and family relationships. You will probably notice that this chapter on therapy is organized differently from the previous chapter. The reason is that therapy tends to be tailored individually based on the needs of the family and the perspective of the therapist. Although some types of therapy are more effective than others, different approaches are effective for different children, teens, and families. The specific objectives of therapy will vary, based on the child's and family's needs and the orientation of the therapist, but the overarching goals of therapy are to improve quality of life, to prevent or reduce the damage that mood disorders can do to relationships (peer and family), and to maximize normal development.

What We Know and What We Don't Know

Empirically validated treatments are types of therapy that have been tested through research with families and children and that have been shown to work. This means that participants in these therapies experienced some improvement—usually lessening of depressive symptoms. For depression, two primary types of therapy have been shown to work— cognitive–behavioral therapy (CBT) and interpersonal therapy (IPT). Cognitive–behavioral therapy involves teaching the relationships among thoughts, feelings, and behavior to improve a child's or teen's ability to manage negative feelings (e.g., sadness, anger, anxiety). Some components of CBT are problem solving, communication skills, anger management, activity scheduling, and cognitive restructuring (i.e., learning to substitute helpful ways of thinking for the hurtful ways of thinking common in depression). CBT has been used successfully with school-age children who report depressive symptoms, as well as with depressed adolescents.

IPT seeks to reduce depressive symptoms and to improve interpersonal functioning by improving communication skills in significant relationships, and it has been used successfully with depressed adolescents.

Family therapy shows significant promise for helping depressed children and teenagers and their families. Family therapy typically involves the child or teen, as well as at least one parent. In many cases, it will involve both parents, possibly siblings, and sometimes extended family members. The goals of family therapy are often to improve communication and problem solving, reduce conflict, and increase positive interactions. Although still in the early stages of research, psychoeducation (providing information, social support, and skill building to patients and families as a way of improving symptom management and family functioning) is also a potentially helpful intervention for children with depression and their families.

Research on therapy for depression, also called *psychosocial treatment,* is significantly ahead of research on bipolar disorder, which is in its very early stages. CBT and psychoeducation both show promise to become empirically validated treatments for bipolar disorder.

So we know that CBT and IPT are effective for treating depression. We also know that family therapy and psychoeducation may also be helpful. For bipolar disorder, CBT and psychoeducation are both promising. There is much that we still don't know and need to learn about psychosocial treatments for mood disorders.

We support empirically validated treatments because there is evidence to suggest that they work. However, not all therapies have been studied carefully, and many therapists incorporate parts of a number of treatment models into their work. If you find a therapist who doesn't work specifically from the models we've outlined in this chapter but who has a good relationship with you and your child and seems to be helpful, stick with him or her. As long as you and your child feel comfortable and therapy is helping, we would not advocate a change. However, if your child loves going to therapy because she likes playing with the toys in her therapist's office but no benefit is apparent, it might be time to rethink the issue. By the same token, a highly recommended therapist working from the best empirically validated treatment is useless if he doesn't connect well with you and your child.

How Therapy Works: The Practical Issues

Parents often don't know what to expect from therapy and fear that they won't make the best choices for their child because they don't know what to look for. To help guide you through this murky territory, we've outlined some general principles to think about as you seek therapy for your child and family.

How Should Sessions Be Structured?

Therapy can be structured in different ways based on who is included in a session: the patient alone (individual therapy), the parent(s) alone (parent guidance), the patient and one or more family member(s) (conjoint or family therapy), or other children who have similar problems or diagnoses (group therapy). Therapy goals vary depending on who's included in a session. Often these different therapy structures are used in combination to meet the needs of a particular child and family.

In general individual therapy for children with mood disorders is used to improve self-esteem, build coping skills, and increase symptom management. Family therapy can be used to improve communication and problem solving, to identify and resolve family conflict, and to improve coping and symptom management skills. Parent guidance is used to help parents cope with difficult aspects of the mood disorder and co-occurring disorders and to develop specific skills and strategies for managing the mood disorder and other family issues. Group therapy can be particularly useful in improving social skills.

When Jeremiah was six years old, he was referred to a child and adolescent psychiatrist by his pediatrician due to violent rages and hypersexual behavior. The psychiatrist started Jeremiah on a mood stabilizer and referred the family to Dr. Smithfield, a psychologist experienced with young children with mood disorders. During the initial phase of therapy, when Jeremiah was still experiencing severe symptoms and was not yet stabilized on medications, the focus of the sessions was crisis and symptom management. Dr. Smithfield spent much of the session time with Jeremiah's mother, Sue (her husband, Ken, was unable to attend most sessions due to his work schedule). During this time Dr. Smithfield helped Sue learn to recognize Jeremiah's symptoms and develop plans for managing his rages and other particularly difficult behaviors. Dr. Smithfield also spent some time with Jeremiah during each session. During this time she was able to observe his symptoms firsthand, learn how Jeremiah talked about his symptoms, and develop a strong relationship with him. She helped Jeremiah learn to label his moods, and together they developed a list of strategies for Jeremiah to try when he felt really angry (such as going out to his sandbox, asking to take a bath, and running around the yard with the family dog).

In Jeremiah's case, Dr. Smithfield started by helping the family learn to cope with their current set of symptoms. In this early phase of therapy with such a young child, the bulk of the time was spent with Jeremiah's mother. In the case of an adolescent, the focus might be on individual therapy instead.

Which Family Members Should Attend?

Like everything else about therapy, there is no hard-and-fast rule about who should be at each session. Who attends therapy should be based on who is needed at sessions and who can reasonably make accommodations to be at sessions. Often only one parent can routinely attend sessions due to work schedule constraints. This can work fine, as long as the parent who attends sessions is able to share session content with the other parent and the parents are generally in agreement about treatment. If there is significant conflict between parents or disagreement about treatment, it may be necessary to shift schedules so that both parents can attend sessions, at least temporarily, or to add a couples' therapist to the mix of treatment providers. There may be times when including siblings or extended family members will be useful. We often invite siblings to join a session or two when the "primary" child or teenager is relatively stable and when issues of parity, severe sibling rivalry, or imitation are a problem (we discuss sibling issues further in Chapter 13). Including extended family members can be very helpful if these extended family members are involved in your child's care.

Who should attend sessions and how each session should be structured (e.g., twenty-five minutes of individual therapy followed by twenty-five minutes of family therapy) are individual decisions made by your therapist in conjunction with you. Such decisions underscore the importance of trusting your therapist, being confident in his or her expertise, and sharing your wishes or concerns with him or her.

What Determines the Focus of Therapy?

The focus of therapy changes based on the status of the illness, on the child's developmental stage, and on current issues or concerns. In addition to helping Jeremiah's parents, Dr. Smithfield began to teach Jeremiah coping strategies. Starting at a very basic level because of his young age, she helped him identify his moods and develop a repertoire of strategies for dealing with his more difficult moods. As he got older and his repertoire of skills grew, Jeremiah was able to understand and take on more responsibility for managing his illness.

By the time Jeremiah was eight, his mood was significantly more stable (a combination of two mood stabilizers and an atypical antipsychotic seemed to be working well), and he was complaining about his lack of friends at school. Still working with Dr. Smithfield, the organization of therapy shifted to more individual therapy time with Jeremiah while continuing to allow some parent guidance and family time. Individual sessions focused on helping Jeremiah learn to interpret and negotiate social situations. Sue played an important role in this process because she often was able to provide more detailed and accurate information about the social situations that Jeremiah described during sessions. In addition, Dr. Smithfield recommended that Jeremiah join an eight-session social skills group. In the group, Jeremiah had the opportunity to practice positive interactions with other children his age. He learned a variety of social skills that he practiced first with group members, then tried at school, reporting back to the group how his new behaviors worked.

At age eight, Jeremiah was more able to maximize his use of individual therapy time. His use of therapy is likely to change many times as he progresses through elementary school and into middle and high school. In some cases, the same therapist can progress with a child into adolescence. In other cases, a shift makes sense. These are decisions you should make with the input of your treatment team and your child or teen.

What Should (and Should Not) Happen in Therapy

Therapy is not a "one size fits all" proposition, and there is probably an exception to every rule that we state, but we have listed here for you some general rules of thumb. These "rules" are meant to help you develop the tools you need to evaluate (or seek) therapy services. As with all things, remember that you are a consumer. Do research, ask questions, and above all else, be an active partner in the process.

Rapport Should Be Strong

Your child or adolescent should feel comfortable spending time with his or her therapist. The relationship between therapist and patient is a critical ingredient for good treatment. However, keep in mind that achieving a good relationship may take some time.

When Krissy (thirteen) came to her first therapy session, everything about her demeanor indicated mistrust and skepticism. She sat with her arms crossed, made minimal eye contact, and made few spontaneous comments except, "I don't know why I'm here." Her new therapist, a young woman, was chosen by Krissy's parents because they thought Krissy would relate best to a young woman. After the first session, Krissy's mother called the therapist, because Krissy wouldn't tell her parents anything about the session except to continue saying, "I don't know why you're making me go." The therapist reassured Krissy's mother that things had gone reasonably well and that Krissy had agreed to come for another session. Although Krissy steadily refused to share session content with her parents, she looked more and more relaxed after each session. The therapist saved two minutes at the end of each session to provide Krissy's mother with some general feedback on how things were going. The therapist also reassured Krissy that she would not share session content but would give general feedback about how Krissy was doing.

Confidentiality Should Be Defined and Maintained

The backbone of therapy is the expectation that what is said during a session is private or confidential. Although confidentiality is important, it has its limits. Krissy's therapist willingly gave her mother feedback on how things were going but did not share specifics of session content. If Krissy had been sharing information that indicated she was in danger (i.e., she was suicidal), her therapist would have shared that information with Krissy's mother so that Krissy's mother could help keep her safe. Teenagers in particular feel very strongly about confidentiality. They are focused (appropriately) on achieving independence from their parents and need to be able to talk with the expectation that what they say will not be shared. Many teenagers are dealing with issues of sexuality and feel very strongly about those discussions not being shared with parents. As the parent of a teenager, you continue to have legal rights to your teen's medical records. However, respecting your teen's privacy and trusting your teen's therapist to give you the information you *do* need may be crucial to your teen's recovery.

Different therapists will handle confidentiality slightly differently. The best thing you can do as a consumer and as a parent is to ask about confidentiality at the initial session. You should know how you will be kept informed about the progress of therapy, as well as what information will be kept confidential and what will be shared. You should know when confidentiality will be broken (e.g., if safety is at risk). You should have a sense of how your child or teen feels about confidentiality. Common expectations make for a smoother relationship. Some children are most comfortable when their parent is in the room, and others talk more openly when alone with a therapist.

Cody is sixteen. He was referred for therapy after being discharged from the hospital, where he was diagnosed with major depression after taking an overdose of his mother's back pain medicine. His mother accompanied him to the initial therapy session with Dr. Patterson, during which Cody barely spoke. After the three met together for fifteen minutes, Dr. Patterson asked to speak with Cody alone. Cody seemed relieved and became significantly more talkative. He explained that he loves his mother but that she gets worried, and when worried, she gets "in his face" too much. Cody's suicide attempt had been precipitated by some problems with his girlfriend, which he felt his parents wouldn't understand. Cody and Dr. Patterson agreed that session content would be kept confidential with the exception that Dr. Patterson would have to let Cody's parents know if he ever felt Cody was in danger. Dr. Patterson agreed to always give Cody the opportunity to share such information with his parents himself before he would speak with them.

Before ending the initial session, Cody's mother joined them again. Dr. Patterson and Cody outlined the confidentiality plan for her. She agreed to the plan and asked if it would be OK if she called Dr. Patterson periodically for general updates. This was fine with both Dr. Patterson and Cody. Dr. Patterson promised to share the content of those phone calls with Cody.

Therapy Should Increase Hopefulness

Experiencing a mood disorder or living with someone with a mood disorder can be overwhelming and can lead to a sense of hopelessness. Therapy, whether individual, family, or parent guidance, should increase hopefulness.

Elizabeth had read every parenting book she could find, had taken a positive parenting class, and had even met with a counselor through her employee assistance program at work. Although her mother and sister had encouraged her to get more help, she had little faith that any doctor could help. Elizabeth was feeling increasingly as though her eight-year-old daughter Maria's problems were all due to her parenting and her divorce four years ago. Maria had become increasingly difficult to manage. Sometimes her energy level was so high that it seemed as though a tornado was going through the house. Maria hadn't been getting to sleep until close to midnight each night, which was causing Elizabeth to get increasingly tired herself. Maria's counselor had encouraged Elizabeth to use time-outs and to be consistent with rewards and consequences. But it didn't seem as though Maria had responded at all. At times Maria would get so angry over what seemed to be nothing that she would start destroying her toys and hitting Elizabeth if she came too close. Elizabeth was on her own with Maria and was feeling hopeless. A friend at work had an eighteen-year-old son who had had similar problems as a child and was now on medication. She gave Elizabeth the name of her son's psychologist. Dr. Henderson evaluated Maria and diagnosed her with bipolar disorder. She told Elizabeth that Maria was likely to need medication and recommended that Maria see a psychiatrist. In the meantime, she started to work with Elizabeth to develop a crisis management plan. Elizabeth was relieved to know that she was not the cause of Maria's problems. With the help of Dr. Henderson, she began to feel empowered to help Maria.

Therapy Should Help Define Problems and Make Them More Manageable

Part of a therapist's role is to help you identify, define, and break down problems into manageable components. In Part I you learned how to recognize your different "piles"—symptoms of the mood disorder, co-occurring disorders, and normal development. As you come to understand your piles, you can develop strategies to cope with each one. Therapy should help you more clearly define your piles and develop plans for managing them. This may mean that some piles are put on the back burner. For example, for a child who overeats and is significantly overweight, one pile might consist of eating habits and weight management. It would be unwise, however, to tackle this pile before achieving a stable mood, as it will not likely be successful. The eating-habits plan might need to wait until the time is right.

When Ronda first sought an evaluation for her ten-year-old son Tyrone, she only knew that things weren't going well. Ronda got at least one call per week from the school, every little thing felt like a battle, and she felt as though she was constantly yelling at Tyrone. To make matters worse, Tyrone was significantly overweight, and his pediatrician had encouraged Ronda to work on getting his weight down by reducing high-fat and sugary foods in his diet.

Ronda was overwhelmed and didn't know where to start. She sought therapy with Dr. Renquist, who had been recommended to her by a friend. After a thorough evaluation Dr. Renquist began to help Ronda define the problems and break them into solvable pieces. He provided a name for the problem: He diagnosed Tyrone with major depression, as well as oppositional defiant disorder (ODD) and ADHD. He also referred Tyrone to a child and adolescent psychiatrist for a medication evaluation.

The next step was to recognize that school was not working well for Tyrone. Dr. Renquist suggested that Tyrone might qualify for and benefit from special education services and suggested that Ronda request a multifactored evaluation through the school (we go into school issues in more detail in Chapter 10).

The third step was to create some opportunities for Ronda and Tyrone to spend positive time together. During one therapy session, Tyrone told his mother that he really liked it when they played board games together. They decided to make Saturday nights their game time. Although Dr. Renquist agreed with Tyrone's pediatrician that reducing his weight was important for his health and self-esteem, he suggested that they wait until some of the other issues were under better control. This reduced the pressure on Ronda and removed one battleground for Ronda and Tyrone.

Through therapy, Ronda began to see specific problem areas with potential solutions rather than being overwhelmed by a global sense of things not going well. Eventually, as Tyrone's performance at school and relationship with his mother began to improve, Ronda gradually began to introduce more healthful snacks and main courses into their diet. She also convinced Tyrone that some of their "Fun Nights" on Saturdays could include going to their local YMCA, where they could swim and work out on the treadmills, and exercise bicycles. Eventually, Tyrone enrolled in a tae kwon do class, in which he experienced success in a physical endeavor—a new experience for Tyrone.

Therapy Should Encourage Growth on the Part of Parents and Children

Therapy should encourage your child to grow and mature and should challenge you as a parent to build a set of skills and a philosophy that will be most helpful to your child. The "usual and customary" parenting techniques often do not work or are insufficient to deal with the problems of children with mood disorders. Mood disorders require significantly more creativity, flexibility, and stick-to-itiveness from parents. Thus working with a professional who has experience with childhood mood disorders can help significantly.

Kathy and Tim are dubious about parent guidance. They know Seth needs help and that *he* needs therapy. Seth has huge screaming fits every time something doesn't go his way and is constantly irritable, so that everyone else in the family walks on eggshells around him. Kathy and Tim have successfully gotten their two older children (now twelve and sixteen) to middle school and high school, respectively. They wonder what a therapist can tell them about how to raise and discipline their nine-year-old son.

Despite their reluctance, they agreed to Dr. Burton's suggestion that they have a few sessions without Seth. Dr. Burton started by asking how parenting Seth was different from parenting their two older children. This led into a discussion about the impact of Seth's mood disorder on family life (Dr. Burton had recently diagnosed Seth with dysthymic disorder and ODD). Dr. Burton helped Kathy and Tim recognize how Seth's mood disorder changes family dynamics. Although they were good parents who worked well together as a team, Seth's needs were different and required a whole new way of approaching parenting and discipline. Because one of the most stressful parts of the day with Seth was right after school, Dr. Burton suggested making an after-school plan to help Seth wind down. In a joint session with Seth and his parents, Dr. Burton helped the family develop an after-school stress-relief plan that started with a snack and ten minutes of Kathy's undivided time, as she listened to Seth tell her about his day. After his snack and chat time, Seth would choose from a list of enjoyable activities that ranged from swinging in the tire swing in the backyard to playing with his Legos.

After two weeks of using the plan, life with Seth seemed to be somewhat better. He was more willing to do his homework after having some time to unwind first. Seth seemed less irritable overall in the evenings. Kathy also found that, if she spent some undivided time with Seth right away, he was less demanding for the rest of the afternoon. At the same time, Dr. Burton worked with Seth on taking more responsibility for his moods. Instead of taking his irritability out on those around him, Dr. Burton encouraged Seth to find things to do and positive ways to think that help him feel better instead of making him and those around him feel worse.

Therapy should always challenge your child or teen to make positive changes. In a nonthreatening and supportive manner, your child's therapist should encourage your child to try new strategies and to take on more and more responsibility.

Elisa, at seven, loved going to therapy. She had been working with her therapist since age five. Her therapist had an office full of toys and games. However, Elisa's parents, Anne and Chris, were getting increasingly frustrated. Elisa was now taking Prozac, and her sleep and appetite problems had improved. She was less irritable, but she was still having tantrums every time she didn't get her way. Despite Anne's repeated descriptions of these tantrums to Elisa's therapist, therapy did not seem to be helping very much. At the beginning of one session, Anne asked the therapist to save some time for her at the end (sessions had been primarily individual from the time Elisa started). Anne asked about Elisa's progress and goals for therapy. After this meeting it was apparent to Anne that the therapist did not have a clear sense of goals for Elisa and was not challenging Elisa to develop new coping skills.

Elisa's parents decided that it was time for a shift. They let Elisa's therapist know that they were going to change therapists and scheduled a good-bye session for Elisa. With Elisa's new therapist, Anne and Chris stayed more involved from the beginning and started with a common set of goals, the first of which was for Elisa to begin to take more responsibility for managing her mood and to find new ways to handle frustration and disappointment instead of throwing tantrums.

Therapy Should Be Nonblaming

There is nothing like blame to make a person feel defeated and demoralized. Therapy should not be a place for the blame game—not for the therapist blaming parents or children, for parents blaming children, for children blaming parents, nor for parents blaming each other. Many parents of children with mood disorders have had the experience of a therapist directly or indirectly blaming them for their child's problems. Although there is no such thing as a perfect parent, we don't know any parents who would wish the ravages of a mood disorder on their child.

When Margo met with Dr. Thomas for the first time, she seemed hesitant and defeated. She described herself as being in desperate need of help managing her son, Michael, who was six. She had been told repeatedly to use behavioral charts, point systems, and even "tough love" to manage his rages, hyperactivity, and sometimes odd behavior (he once took off all of his clothes and ran down the street screaming, "I'm king of the world!"). Dr. Thomas listened to her describe Michael's behavior and the various strategies that had been suggested to her. Next, she asked Margo to wipe the slate clean. Dr. Thomas then told Margo that what she described sounded like the symptoms of a manic episode and that Michael sounded like he had bipolar disorder. She asked Margo to start thinking in terms of Michael's symptoms rather than his behavioral problems. Dr. Thomas stressed the importance of Michael's seeing a child and adolescent psychiatrist for a medication evaluation as soon as possible and referred Margo to a psychiatrist in her practice. Margo left the initial session feeling reenergized. For the first time, Michael's problems seemed fixable.

Dr. Thomas did several helpful things. First, she let Margo know that her parenting strategies had not caused Michael's problems, and, furthermore, that excellent parenting techniques alone would not fix Michael's problems. Second, by labeling Michael's problems as symptoms, she immediately named Michael's mood disorder as the enemy (see our "Naming the Enemy" exercise in Chapter 2). Blame is almost always unhelpful and damaging, whether it is the therapist blaming a family member or one family member blaming another.

When Cindy brought her four-year-old son, Travis, in to be evaluated, she was well prepared. She had done extensive reading and was now convinced that Travis had bipolar disorder. She was able to clearly describe his current symptoms, his developmental history, and everything they had already tried. Cindy had drawn their family tree and had mapped out an extensive history of mood disorders on Travis's father's side of the family. Cindy clearly believed that Travis had inherited bipolar disorder from his father's side of the family. The psychologist, Dr. Lind, stopped Cindy and commended her for how well she had prepared for the evaluation. Dr. Lind asked if Travis had some positive traits that were like his father's. Cindy smiled and talked about how much they look alike and how athletic Travis is, just like his father. Dr. Lind explained that although the family tree is helpful in understanding Travis and his illness, it can be damaging if it is used to blame one parent. No parent would ever choose to give bipolar disorder to a child.

Therapy Should Do No Harm (or, If Necessary, Quit While You're Ahead)

Therapy should be tailored to a child's developmental stage and current needs. Sometimes it makes the most sense to stop trying rather than making a child resent or hate something that he may find more helpful at a later point in his life.

Benjamin, an eleven-year-old with MDD and ADHD, was referred for therapy by his psychiatrist. Benjamin was doing better at school ‘nce starting a combination of Prozac and Concerta, but he continued to argumentative and challenging at home. Benjamin came for an initial ‘py session along with his mother. The therapist started by meeting with Benjamin. He answered the therapist's questions willingly but with one-word answers, no matter how open ended the question. After meeting with Benjamin, the therapist met alone with Benjamin's mother. During this time, Benjamin interrupted frequently by knocking on the door. Meeting in a conjoint session was equally unproductive, as Benjamin was silly and disruptive. After several sessions, Benjamin's mother reported to their therapist that Benjamin complained constantly about coming and behaved worse on the afternoons on which therapy was scheduled. She and the therapist made a joint decision to shift to working together in parent guidance. They based this decision on knowing that Benjamin's mother was desperate for new ideas to try with Benjamin, that his younger brother and sister were starting in with "copycat" behavior, and that Benjamin did not seem to be benefiting from either individual or conjoint therapy. Benjamin's mother and the therapist agreed to revisit the idea of therapy for Benjamin at a later date.

When Benjamin was fourteen, he agreed to initiate therapy after he became stymied by some complicated peer issues. At that time, Benjamin developed a strong relationship with his new therapist, a colleague of the therapist who had provided episodic parent guidance to his mother. Now that Benjamin was older, he found it very helpful to have someone outside his family help him solve problems with some difficult emotions and relationships.

The Therapist Should Be Suited to Your Child and You

Therapists are human, and they vary in all sorts of ways—their sense of humor, interests, communication style, gender, appearance, and ethnicity. What matters most is that you find a therapist who makes both you and your child feel comfortable, whom you and your child both trust, and who can help your child build a set of skills to help her cope. Your child may be best suited to a therapist with a silly sense of humor and a familiarity with sports. Your adolescent may prefer a therapist who is up on the latest music and is very laid back.

Kayla is a quiet ten-year-old who is often sad and worried. Kayla was willing, and even eager, to start therapy, because she had found her few meetings with the school guidance counselor (a young woman) very helpful. Kayla's mother made an appointment with a child psychologist on their provider list. After meeting with this therapist twice, Kayla asked to switch because he was "too stuffy." Kayla told her mother that she wanted someone who would "get" her. Because Kayla had seemed to relate well to her guidance counselor, her mother called their pediatrician hoping for help in finding the right therapist for Kayla. The pediatrician suggested a call to a local practice with several different child therapists. Kayla's mother described Kayla to the intake person, who suggested a young, soft-spoken female social worker who is also athletic (Kayla is a good athlete and plays soccer, basketball, and softball).

You Should Get Enough but Not Too Much

Although some general guidelines exist, there is no rule about how often therapy should occur. Sometimes when symptoms are severe, sessions are scheduled for more than once a week as a way of preventing the need for hospitalization. In other situations, therapy sessions scheduled sporadically can be very effective (e.g., for a child who is doing very well but just needs to check in periodically).

Justin, who is twelve, was diagnosed with major depression four months ago. He has been doing very well over the past six weeks. He came for his weekly therapy session looking significantly more fidgety than usual. Justin kept looking at his watch and glancing out the window. After fifteen minutes of this out-of-character behavior, Justin's therapist asked him what was going on. Justin grinned sheepishly and told his therapist that his friends were going to go riding on their scooters at 4:00 P.M. and that he wanted to be home in time to join them.

Justin is doing well. His mood has stabilized, and his peer relationships have improved significantly. He is doing so well that his weekly therapy sessions are beginning to interfere with his newly developed friendships. It's time to cut back on session frequency. We want therapy to maximize a child's chances of engaging in age-appropriate activities, not interfere with them. On the other hand, therapy can also be underused. Abigail is a seven-year-old with double depression (dysthymic disorder and major depression). Abigail's family cancels sessions frequently and attends only about once per month. Her mother is overwhelmed by Abigail's needs and feels hopeless. They are typically in the midst of a crisis whenever they attend a session, and therapy does not seem to be helping. Because Abigail has not met frequently with her therapist (sessions are usually predominated by mother's one-on-one time with the therapist in a crisis-management mode), she does not feel very attached to her. Abigail's family is underusing therapy. They have attended therapy so infrequently that they are never able to get past crisis management and into making progress in treatment.

Although there is no set formula for how often therapy sessions should occur, early in treatment regular sessions are probably necessary to make progress. The best rule of thumb is to reevaluate periodically. Talk with your therapist. If you have financial limitations that affect how often you can afford sessions, be realistic about that and share that information with your therapist so she can make realistic plans with you. Review progress and goals. Talk about the frequency of sessions. If session frequency feels burdensome, think about why. Is it because you don't need as much as you're getting or because your life is so stressful that going to therapy just feels like the last straw? If you and the therapist agree that the current frequency is necessary, can you simplify your life so that therapy feels more manageable?

Establishing Treatment Goals

Above all else, therapy should be helpful and should lead to positive changes. Having realistic and mutually agreed-on goals can significantly improve your ability to assess the helpfulness of therapy and maximize its usefulness. Depending on the severity of your child's symptoms, the age of your child, and the status of other interventions (e.g., medication management, school services), treatment goals will vary. Therapy goals should shift over time, from working toward stability when symptoms are acute (and/or severe) to working on maximizing functioning at home, at school, and with peers when symptoms are improving and, finally, to fine-tuning when symptoms are waning. Jeremiah started therapy just as medications were being started. He needed to be stabilized. As stabilization was achieved, the focus of therapy shifted to maximizing his functioning at home and especially with peers. Once he was able to do well at home and at school and had some positive peer relationships, the focus shifted again to fine-tuning (e.g., increasing Jeremiah's personal responsibility for his moods, decreasing his reliance on family members to accommodate his needs). You and your therapist should have a sense of where you are in the goals hierarchy.

When Should We Shift Goals?

Some therapy goals will shift due to changes in the illness itself, whereas other shifts will result from developmental and situational changes.

Samantha started therapy when she was fourteen and had just begun her freshman year in high school. Samantha had become very unhappy as a result of social problems at school. Initially, Samantha used individual therapy to help her develop skills to deal with the social pressures she was experiencing. As Samantha became more comfortable at school and developed a stronger social network, her depressive symptoms diminished. When Samantha's therapist suggested that maybe it was time to discontinue therapy because she was doing so well, Samantha resisted. Her therapist suggested that they use a session to review the goals of therapy. During this session it became clear that although Samantha was feeling better about her peer relationships, she was struggling with her relationship with her parents. Samantha and her therapist decided to invite Samantha's parents to join therapy and to shift the focus of therapy to family relationships.

When a change in functioning occurs (e.g., a reduction or increase in symptoms), therapy goals may shift back to the acute phase of managing symptoms or crises, to maximizing functioning, or to fine-tuning. The direction and nature of therapy also changes when a developmental shift, such as reaching adolescence occurs.

Therapy Should Be Geared to the Severity of the Mood Disorder and the Child/Teen's Level of Functioning

A child who has never experienced a full mood episode but who has a strong family history of mood disorders and tends to have a "fragile" mood may benefit significantly from therapy aimed at increasing her ability to self-regulate and develop coping mechanisms. A teenager with a severe mood disorder will have significantly different therapy needs.

Brandon, our fifteen-year-old with severe depression who ultimately benefited from electroconvulsive therapy (ECT), worked closely with his therapist. Following ECT, Brandon did remarkably better. He began getting A's in school and redeveloping his peer network. However, Brandon came to one therapy session seeming really down. As the session progressed, Brandon explained that he was sure he would never be able to get into college and that he was a complete failure. Because of his worry about college (still a year and a half away), Brandon had not left the house for three days. His therapist first focused on how his behavior was influenced by his mood and, conversely, how his mood was influenced by his behavior. Not leaving the house meant that Brandon had not exercised or participated in any fun activities. This made his mood worse. The therapist and Brandon started by making a list of activities for Brandon to engage in over the next several days. Then they focused on Brandon's thought process. In his description of what was going on, Brandon used words such as *never* and *complete failure*. These words make problems seem permanent and absolute. During the session Brandon and his therapist also developed a different way of talking about Brandon's college concerns (e.g., "I'm worried that my grades won't allow me to go to the college of my dreams, but I should be able to get in to a college that will meet my needs").

Therapy needs vary among children because they all have different temperaments, because they are at different developmental stages, because stressors are unique to each individual, and because each child's mood disorder progresses differently. The *who* (Who is the therapist? Who attends?), *what* (What are the goals? What are the specific strategies?), and *when* (When does therapy happen? How often?) of therapy vary from individual to individual, depending on child and family needs. The bottom line is that therapy should be helpful.

Part III

Helping Your Child Cope

By reading Parts I and II thoroughly, you've laid a critical foundation for helping your child. You now have a solid understanding of the complexity of mood symptoms and syndromes, and you know how to get the most from available treatments. The next step is to build on your foundation by learning strategies that will help steer your child successfully through daily life at home, at school, and wherever else she needs to function.

In Chapter 8, we review some core concepts that, when integrated into day-to-day family life, can make future challenges more manageable. Getting your child to become part of the solution is critical for success, however, so Chapter 9 teaches some specific skills your child can use, the very techniques we teach in our groups and with individual families.

A huge portion of a child's day is spent at school, so in Chapter 10 we show how you can partner with your child and the school system to deal with the kinds of academic and social problems children tend to have as a result of their mood symptoms.

Unfortunately, crises are a common event for families with children who are mood impaired. Although not all of the situations we address in Chapter 11 will be applicable to your family, we hope this chapter serves as a useful reference for you should you need it now or in the future.

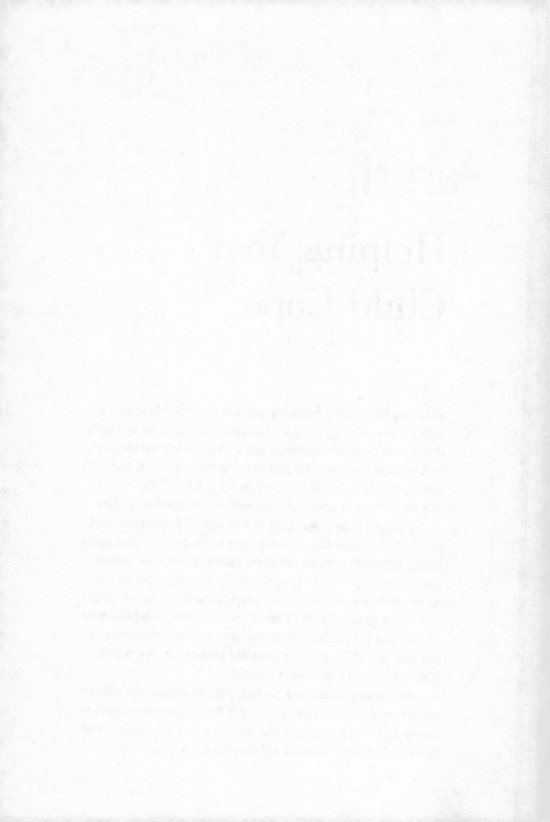

8 Ten Principles for Managing a Mood Disorder

When Rosalita, the oldest of three children, was first seen in therapy at age eight, her parents had already begun to feel demoralized and guilty about their inability to manage Rosalita's behavior. Rosalita had significant difficulty getting along with peers and was frequently irritable at home, and some of the mental health and school professionals that her parents had consulted had insinuated that their parenting strategies were to blame. As Rosalita's parents both came from families in which people did not speak of mental illness, they were not aware of any family history of mood disorders. We've seen this happen with many families: The "ostrich" effect—if no one talks about their family's problems, maybe they will all go away—can easily occur. The problem is, it gets in the way of good care for the child.

It was only after Rosalita experienced a major depressive episode and then started exhibiting manic symptoms that her parents took a new look at their family history. Now that their daughter's symptom profile looked more and more like bipolar disorder, they began to realize that relatives on both sides of their family had also experienced mood problems. Seeing these connections made Rosalita's parents more accepting of her problems. Now, instead of second-guessing their own parenting strategies and responses to Rosalita's often difficult behavior, they started participating more actively in her treatment. With Rosalita's therapist as their coach, Rosalita's parents began to plan proactively how they would manage her symptoms at home. They also set up a meeting with the school to develop strategies to help Rosalita function successfully there. Perhaps most important, with guidance from her therapist, Rosalita's parents began to make a concerted effort to help Rosalita understand that the problems she was facing—keeping her temper in check, saying and doing outrageous things, having difficulty falling asleep, and her loud, intrusive style of talking—were not her fault but rather were all a part of her mood disorder. They also told her she would be a central part of the solution. Rosalita, her parents, Rosalita's psychiatrist, and their therapist began to see themselves as part of the same team that would work together to manage these symptoms.

1. Shrug Off Self-Blame and Take Action

As we stated unequivocally in Chapter 3, blaming yourself for your child's mood problems is counterproductive, wasting time and energy that you could be spending on really helping your child. Once they have you in their grip, self-blame and guilt can blind you to the origins of your child's problems; they can even keep you from seeing the problem in the first place, as in the case of eleven-year-old Latisha. Latisha seemed sad and withdrawn for nine months, starting when her mother abruptly moved out and initiated divorce proceedings. Because her father, Jim, didn't know how to explain the divorce to his daughter, he just let Latisha mope quietly in her bedroom. It wasn't until her grades plummeted and he realized that his daughter wasn't adjusting to the divorce with time that Latisha's father finally took his daughter for an evaluation. After diagnosing Latisha with an adjustment disorder with depressed mood, the psychologist suggested that therapy might be helpful and that Jim be involved. Getting this diagnosis helped Jim realize that Latisha's unhappiness was a real problem and that he needed to take charge. Latisha's psychologist suggested that Jim and Latisha pick at least one fun activity to do together each weekend and that they reorganize their dinner hour so that they would work together in the kitchen. Because Latisha's mom had been the family cook, Latisha and her dad had been eating haphazardly, and often separately, after she departed. Initiating a new tradition in the kitchen allowed Latisha and Jim to reconnect and establish new traditions for their new family structure.

So we repeat: Your child's mood problem isn't your fault, but it is your challenge, and this principle applies not just to getting your child diagnosed and treated, as we discussed in Parts I and II of this book, but also to helping your child develop coping skills for use in daily life.

2. Be Realistic

Learning how to set expectations that are neither too low nor too high for a mood-impaired child can be difficult. We recommend to parents that they use their clinician as a guide to help them determine what to expect of their recovering child and when they should revise expectations. Because mood disorders naturally vacillate in severity (see Figure 1 in Chapter 2), knowing when to expect what from a recovering child is no easy feat.

Twelve-year-old Nick was hospitalized after threatening his ten-year-old sister Karen with a knife during a rage. While in the hospital, an atypical antipsychotic was added to his regimen of Depakote, Trazodone, and Concerta. Although Nick was somewhat better following his hospitalization, he was still very irritable and explosive. Nick and Karen had often fought over whose turn it was to feed, walk, or clean up after their dog, chores they had always shared. So when Nick got home, his mother, Allison, decided to remove the issue by asking Karen if she would accept extra allowance for doing double duty with the dog. This

---

TIPS FOR PARENTS: HOW DO YOU DECREASE EXPECTATIONS TEMPORARILY WITHOUT BABYING YOUR CHILD?

1. Downshift expectations when your child is consistently unable to meet them (persistent failure isn't good for anyone's self-esteem).

2. Raise expectations gradually and evaluate how new expectations are handled.

3. Prioritize.

   a. Make a list of your child's responsibilities, including areas such as self-care, schoolwork, household responsibilities, and behavior toward others.

   b. Start with the most important items on the list (completing homework should come before making the bed). Think creatively about how tasks can gradually become more difficult (e.g., completing homework with assistance may lead to completing homework independently).

4. Acknowledge that your child has an illness from which he or she needs to recover.

removed a source of conflict and helped to smooth Nick's transition back to home. Karen was happy to earn the extra money and looked forward to some special one-on-one time with her mother, who also promised to take her shopping once the extra allowance had accumulated.

Allison also worked with Nick's teachers to reduce his workload temporarily so that he would not have homework when he first returned to school. As Nick's mood improved, his mother began to raise her expectations for her son at home by giving him new chores. Initially, Allison backed off if she met resistance from Nick. Gradually, however, she became more insistent that Nick take on his part of the responsibility. Nick's teachers also began to increase his workload until he was doing the same work as the rest of his class.

Although children need clear and consistent expectations, there are times that expectations need to be adjusted. During a severe mood episode is not the time to insist that your child complete all of her chores. However, as treatment progresses and your child's mood stabilizes, expectations can be increased.

3. Don't Over- or Underregulate

Children need rules to help them regulate their behavior, but too many or too few rules can be a problem.

Tyler is ten. He was diagnosed with dysthymic disorder (DD) six months ago. Tyler is expected to make his bed daily, keep his room picked up, complete his homework independently when he gets home, and unload the dishwasher each day. Tyler's allowance is docked if he has to be reminded to do any of his chores and if he leaves any of his toys on the floor by bedtime. Tyler has frequent conflicts with his parents about toys not being put away and about the way he treats his younger siblings. He frequently feels defeated and frustrated because he finds himself being yelled at when he thinks he is doing OK.

On the other hand, Maggie is eight, and she rules the roost. She was also diagnosed with DD six months ago. Maggie's mother, a single parent, has always found it easier to give in to Maggie's demands than to risk precipitating a tantrum. Maggie cries and screams at her mother when asked to help out around the house, and homework is usually a two-hour marathon session, characterized by Maggie's mom cajoling her to complete each and every spelling word and math problem.

When households have too many rules, children can easily become demoralized. They may either give up trying to please their parents and incorporate an identity as a rule breaker or constantly try to please their parents, rarely meeting with success. Conversely, when households have too few rules or unclear rules, enforcement is impossible, and behavior tends to become out of control. Although this is true for all children, the stakes are higher if your child has a baseline difficulty with managing frustrating situations. Rules should emphasize physical and emotional safety for all family members first. Consequences for breaking rules should be clear and consistent.

4. Keep It Simple

If you're struggling over a particular rule with your child, ask yourself why the rule exists: Is there a good reason for it, or is it arbitrary? Because children with mood disorders may need assistance in a variety of arenas, you (and your child) may start to feel overwhelmed by the numbers of situations you have to address. What to do? Simplify! Write out the list of rules you expect your child to follow. Can you simplify the list to a few basic rules, such as, "No hurting others with your body" and "No hurting others with your words"? Our motto is "simplify, simplify, simplify." You'll be better equipped to be consistent, and your child will do a better job of following rules if he isn't overwhelmed by their complexity.

5. Be Flexible

Your child has a disorder, the symptoms of which do not stay the same day after day. By definition, her functioning will shift over time. As a result, there may be times, especially during severe mood episodes, that some rules get suspended. Although limits on time spent with TV, computers, and video games are generally important for parents to establish and maintain, some flexibility may benefit your child, depending on his phase of illness. A severely depressed teen may reasonably make watching a funny movie part of a plan to increase pleasurable activities. Or a child with severely impaired social skills and no peer group may benefit from spending some time learning to play a particularly popular video game as a way to build common interest with peers. The key is *flexibility*. Is what you are doing working for your child? If it is, great. If not, step back and reevaluate.

6. Choose Your Battles

Parents raising children with mood disorders sometimes describe their situation as "living in a war zone," and many report feeling that they are constantly "walking on eggshells." In either case, the stress of constant "war" or constant tiptoeing is wearing. To minimize the struggles and reduce overall tension, we encourage you to pick your battles. That way your family can find some peace between conflicts.

Eric is twelve and has bipolar disorder. He is an extremely picky eater. Dinnertime frequently ends with Eric having a screaming fit. After many months of miserable dinners, Eric's parents sat down to talk about the problem with him. Eric's primary complaint was that he didn't like most of their regular dinner menus. His mother's primary concerns were that he eat a balanced diet and that he not make a big mess in the kitchen. After some discussion they agreed that Eric could make an alternative meal for himself. The meal would have to include at least one source of protein, one fruit, and one vegetable. His alternate meals could not involve any extra cooking. Eric and his mom made a list of some food choices he could easily prepare, such as peanut butter sandwiches, carrot and celery sticks, and yogurt with fruit, and posted the list on the refrigerator.

Some battles are not worth fighting. If you have a consistent battlefront with your child, think about why. Can you opt out? If there isn't a health or safety reason, you may be able to choose to drop a battle or find a compromise. Compromises should always maintain everyone's physical and emotional health and safety.

Battles over food are particularly good to avoid. No child will starve in a house with food available, and most children could probably benefit from taking a multivitamin regularly anyway. However, some children with mood disorders will also have eating disorders (see Chapter 4). If your child is preoccupied with issues related to weight and food or if your child is underweight or overweight, seek advice from your pediatrician or family doctor and your mental health team. For children and ado-

SHOULD WE PROTECT OUR CHILDREN FROM BAD NEWS?

The answer is yes and no. You should not keep secrets from your child. He is likely to find out or sense that something is wrong. But you can protect your child by talking to him in an age-appropriate manner and at a time when he is able to think about and process the information (i.e., not just before he leaves for school or right before he goes to bed). Also, you can choose to have ongoing discussions about the matter (e.g., with your spouse or other friends or family members) in a more private setting. If an upsetting event is coming in the future, you might consider the best time to tell your child. Some children do better with time to adjust prior to the event, whereas others brood, worry, or act out in response to knowing something is coming. Consider the age of your child and her temperament to determine how and when to share upsetting news. We typically recommend providing a short explanation, then answering questions your child raises. This way you provide the information your child is seeking without going into detail beyond what your child wants or needs to know. Several days later you can ask your child if she has more questions. This process allows the child to obtain just enough information, without being bombarded with too much information that she is not equipped to handle.

lescents who are overweight or who have particularly poor eating habits, consider working with a nutritionist or registered dietician experienced in working with children. Children and adolescents may do a better job of improving their eating habits if food is removed from the battleground.

7. Become Expert Problem Solvers

You've learned a lot about your child's disorder. We encourage you to use that knowledge to develop new strategies to manage the symptoms. You may be able to do this on your own, or you may find that consulting with your therapist will give you some fresh ideas to try.

Becky is fourteen and was diagnosed with bipolar disorder and obsessive–compulsive disorder (OCD) when she was nine. Despite some adjustments to her medications, Becky continues to have very difficult mornings. She wakes up in an irritable mood and has extreme difficulty choosing an outfit to wear. Becky tries multiple combinations, finds something unacceptable about each one, then insists she has to change her whole outfit, including her undergarments. During Becky's outfit-choosing process, she asks her mother, Amy, again and again for reassurance, to the point that

Amy cannot get ready for work and is frequently late. Many mornings end with both Becky and Amy angry and sometimes crying. Becky's father, Bill, makes attempts to reassure Becky but is relatively uninvolved in the morning dilemmas.

We recommend that you think of this dilemma and others like it as reflections of the child's symptoms. Then, turning to your family's communication and problem-solving skills, think of ways to manage the symptom. If a problem has a potential solution, it instantly seems less overwhelming. Start by defining the problem. Be specific and define it from different family members' points of view.

What Is the Problem?

Becky's perspective: Becky hates mornings. As soon as she wakes up, she can't stop thinking about what to wear and how none of her clothes seem "right." She hates even more how she and her mom get into fights over getting dressed nearly every day.

Mom's perspective: Amy wants to reassure and help Becky but feels rejected and frustrated when her reassurance and assistance don't make her daughter feel better. Amy is also encountering problems at work because she arrives late and frazzled.

Who Needs to Know about It?

Becky and her parents are aware of the problem and need to begin tackling it. Her prescribing physician needs to know about the ongoing morning irritability. Becky's therapist should also be part of the problem-solving process (until the family becomes skilled enough to address these problems independently). If Becky is arriving at school frustrated and frazzled, just like her mother, it might be helpful for Becky's teachers to know a little about the problem and to be reassured that the family is working toward a solution. And Becky needs to understand the role of her mood in making mornings so difficult. The more she understands about how her morning mood affects her ability to get dressed and get her day started, the better able she will be to help herself.

Next, the family members involved with the problem should brainstorm a list of possible solutions. Before judging each suggestion's merit, Becky, Amy, and Bill should sit down together to name as many possible solutions as they can generate.

What Are Possible Solutions?

- *Becky:* Choose and try on outfits the night before.
- *Bill:* Increase Becky's coping skills so that she can be more self-reliant in the mornings.
- *Amy:* Use therapy to deal with related issues, such as body image concerns and concerns about fitting in socially.
- *Amy:* Have Dad be responsible for getting Becky to school each day.
- *Bill:* Send Mom out of Becky's room.
- *Bill:* Adjust medications further.

Next, Becky, Bill, and Amy should weigh the pros and cons for each of their ideas.

What Are Their Pros and Cons?

- Choosing outfits the night before may be helpful because Becky is more able to resist obsessive thoughts in the evenings (mornings are her hardest time). The problem may be that even if she chooses the night before, Becky still may find problems with outfits the next morning. She would need some strategies to use to resist those thoughts.
- Becky has been working hard in therapy and has been making quite a few gains. She agrees that talking with her therapist to develop more strategies is a really good idea. However, she snaps at Mom for suggesting that any of this conflict is over her not liking her own appearance—she says it is all about the clothes, not her body.
- Getting Dad more involved may help—we don't really know what would happen. He has thus far been out of the fracas.
- Mom and Becky have been having very difficult morning interactions. Reducing her involvement might help improve their relationship. Also, Becky seems to seek more and more reassurance when it's available. Because Mom can be very helpful in getting outfits put together, this problem might be dealt with by having Mom help Becky the previous evening.
- Adjusting Becky's medications may help reduce her obsessive thinking in the mornings. She is taking Luvox to manage her OCD. With the exception of this morning wardrobe issue, the

Luvox has been very helpful. The last time Becky's psychiatrist tried increasing her dose, Becky became hypomanic. Depending on her current blood level of Depakote, another possibility would be to increase Becky's mood stabilizer to further decrease her irritability.

Next, Becky, Amy, and Bill need to decide which strategy to try first.

Pick One and Try It!

With the help of Becky's therapist, the family made a plan. Becky would consult with her mother about potential outfits, then Becky would choose, try on, and lay out an outfit the night before. Becky agreed to get dressed as soon as she got up. Further, she would not look at herself in the mirror. The plan allowed Becky to ask once if the outfit looked OK.

At the same time, Becky would work with her therapist to gain some insight into why there has been so much conflict over getting dressed. They might focus on ways to manage her obsessional thinking, as well as why she is so concerned about looking a certain way. They might also examine why she needs so much reassurance from her mother and how she can begin to become more independent (an appropriate goal for a fourteen-year-old).

After following through with a solution, the family needs to step back and evaluate the relative success of their plan. If your first solution works, do it again. If it doesn't work, pick a different solution and try that next.

How Did It Work?

Becky and her family tried the plan. It worked for the first two days, but by the third day Becky became "stuck" in front of the mirror. The conflictual mornings returned.

Try Again

After their first plan backfired, Becky's family met again with their therapist to devise a second plan. They decided that Amy should request a change in her work schedule (her company encourages flextime to maintain company morale) so that her new hours would be 7:00 A.M. to 3:00 P.M. instead of 8:30 A.M. to 4:30 P.M. This change would mean that Amy would provide some support for Becky in the evening but would try to phase out her involvement in Becky's clothing choice. Amy would then leave for work before Becky got up in the morning. They also decided to increase Becky's individual therapy time until the "dressing dilemma" was resolved. Because Becky was not accustomed to asking her dad for reassurance, Becky began to tackle getting dressed more independently. She began using strategies that she and her therapist devised and gradually became able to put on an outfit that she had chosen the night before, eat breakfast, and head out the door with only minor concerns about her outfit. The benefit for Becky and the rest of the family was that Mom now came home thirty minutes before Becky and her brother got home from school. Her newly available time during the after-school hours further helped to reduce the overall stress in the family.

**FAMILY EXERCISE 4:
SYMPTOM MANAGEMENT USING
PROBLEM SOLVING**

- For this project you (and your spouse or partner) and your child should identify a problem in the family that may revolve around one of your child's symptoms (e.g., after-school irritability leading to sibling conflict).
- Both (all) of you should identify who should be involved in the discussion about the problem.
- As a group, brainstorm possible solutions to the problem.
- Next, think about the pros and cons of each solution and pick the best solution (the one with the most pros).
- Finally, try the solution to the problem that you've picked.
- Evaluate whether it works (you might make some notes in a journal during the time that you're trying the new solution). If it doesn't work, go back to your solution list and pick the next best solution to try next.

8. Be Good Communicators

Talking to kids with mood disorders can be challenging. When your child is feeling upset, your natural instinct may be to soothe and reassure. When your child has a problem, your parental instinct is most likely to fix it. These instincts, although important, can lead you down the wrong path for effective communication with your child. As you read through the following list, you may be struck by the fact that these tips are useful in communicating with anyone, not only with a child who has a mood disorder. What we find in our work with families is that excellent communication is good for everyone but that children with special needs (such as mood disorders) have an extra-special need for good communication.

Here are some rules of thumb to help you communicate better with your child.

- *Listen to, without "correcting," your child's feelings and concerns.* As you listen to your child describe how a peer was mean to her and how sad she is about it, let her be sad and provide support. We encourage parents to visualize themselves holding a container for this job—it may be a handcrafted pottery bowl, a tight, plastic-sealed storage container, or a great big bucket. Your first job, as a parent, is to let your child pour his feelings into your container. Working on solving problems comes only after you have acknowledged and validated your child's feelings. Try asking questions to understand your child better (e.g., "How did you feel about that?"), acknowledging that you are hearing your child (e.g., "Wow, it sounds like you felt really sad when that happened!") or making supportive comments (e.g., "I'm sorry that happened to you").
- *Ask if your child wants suggestions before giving advice.* Jumping in with ways to fix your child's problems before your child is ready for help can lead to friction in your relationship. If your child isn't ready for advice, he might discard your ideas out of hand, which may lead you to feel rejected and frustrated. On the other hand, if you ask first, your child is more likely to listen to your ideas and feel that you are validating his concerns and supporting him. He is also more likely to actively partner with you in problem solving if he is invited into the process rather than given the solution.
- *Talk directly with your child about matters that concern you, but choose your battles.* Talking with your child directly about situations or behaviors that concern you can help lead to better problem solving. However, if you share too many concerns too frequently, your child will feel criticized. Depressed children are already demoralized, and research has clearly demonstrated that critical interactions make the course of depression worse, not better. If you get in the habit of choosing only important issues, you will also avoid arguments over less meaningful things. For example, you might choose to discuss your concerns about your teen's habit of staying up until 3:00 or 4:00 in the morning on Friday and Saturday nights because you fear that she might trigger another mood episode. This is an important health issue. We know that good sleep habits are an important part of managing a mood disorder. On the other hand, whether or not your daughter practices her clarinet daily may not be an issue worth raising. Ultimately, your teen will suffer the consequences of not practicing enough, but this is not life threatening.

• *Address issues when they're small instead of letting them build up.* Over the six months following his inpatient hospitalization, Nick gradually returned to his responsibilities at home and school. After a few months of things going fairly well, his mother noticed that Nick and his sister Karen were beginning to fight more frequently. Unsure of the root of the problem, she brought up the issue at their next family therapy session. During that session it came out that Karen resented the extra support and attention Nick had been getting. Karen and her mother agreed to have a special girls' day out every other weekend. With that plan instituted, peace was restored in the household (although, like normal siblings, Nick and Karen still squabble sometimes). Because Nick's mother noticed and addressed the increase in fighting early, she was able to avoid a buildup of tension in the family and the probability that Nick would be blamed for any problems that occurred. When problems are caught early, they carry less emotional weight, cause fewer conflicts, and are generally easier to manage. Again, modeling a calm, matter-of-fact way of solving problems is very important for your child, who needs to learn this skill to manage her symptoms.

• *Emphasize the positive.* Remember to give praise and positive feedback whenever it is legitimate. Improvement occurs gradually and is greatly facilitated by having someone notice the small improvements made. Depressed people are programmed to overfocus on negative comments about themselves, the world around them, and the future. Providing realistic positive feedback (not just sunny phrases with no support, such as "It's OK, honey, everything will work out") helps to counteract this drift toward the negative. For example, after Nick had been home from the hospital for one and a half weeks, he began helping out inconsistently with family chores. Although he still wasn't back to routinely completing his previous list of chores, Nick was doing more than he had been prior to hospitalization. His mother praised him for what he was doing, and that encouraged Nick to do more.

• *Give negative feedback in a calm voice.* A calm voice will help keep the focus of the criticism on the action (or lack of action) rather than on your child as a person. When you ask your child to do something differently, try to make positive requests for change and remember your "XYZ's" (that is, "When you do X, I feel Y, and I would like you to do Z"). For example, instead of yelling "STOP YELLING AT ME!" to your child, say, "When you yell at me while you are standing right next to me, it hurts my ears and I feel angry. I would like you to talk more softly." You will probably need to give yourself a time-out or a break from the situation until you are very well practiced in this in order to keep your cool! Once you've mastered the ability to stay calm yourself, you are also modeling highly effective communication to your child. After all, yelling at your child to get him to stop yelling doesn't make much sense when you stop to think about it.

We do recognize the incredible frustration you must feel when you get into these tense situations—in Chapter 14 we talk about how to deal with your own feelings in all of this—and that is no small consideration.

• *Make more positive than negative comments.* Constructive criticism is a great way to help someone grow and change *as long as* only a little criticism is delivered at a time. Research has shown that it takes seven positive comments to counteract a negative comment. So make it a point to make more positive than critical comments to your child each day. This sounds easy, but it isn't! Try this exercise to "get in shape." In the morning, put twenty pennies in your left pocket. Each time you praise your child, move one penny to your right pocket. Each time you criticize, move a penny from your right pocket back to your left pocket. Try to have all of the pennies transferred from the left to the right pocket by the end of the day.

• *Remember the power of your body language.* You may be saying more with your body than you do with words. A tense face, clenched hands, and stern-looking stance—what we call *nonverbal communication*—adds a mixed message to any positive words coming out of your mouth. Your nonverbal communication and tone of voice will significantly influence the response you get. And, just as with the other pointers we've been sharing, as you master this lesson and use it in interacting with your child, you will also be modeling healthy communication to him. Just as your child will benefit from seeing your nonverbal communication match your verbal communication, so will you appreciate it when his nonverbal language can match his verbal interchanges.

• *Avoid playing "Twenty Questions."* As a parent, anxiety can easily get the best of you. Don't, however, continually quiz your child about how she's feeling as a way to monitor her. Research has clearly demonstrated that an intrusive interaction style (while we doubt that is your intention, it is probably how your child experiences it) slows down recovery for children who are depressed. Additionally, if your child is afraid to "give you an inch or you'll take a mile," she'll probably be less likely to open up to you when she really needs your advice.

9. Name the Enemy

Be sure to differentiate your child's personality, characteristics, strengths, and weaknesses from your child's illness and symptoms. Review the "Naming the Enemy" exercise periodically (see Chapter 2). Recognizing irritability as a symptom, rather than as one of your child's traits, can help you maintain a more positive relationship with your child.

10. Share the Joy and the Pain

Establish a shared understanding with your parenting partner. Having a parenting partner who has a similar understanding of your child's illness and the importance of his treatment can be a lifesaver. When parents work together, extremely difficult situations can become manageable. When parents work against each other, the opposite is true.

In some cases parents can easily find common ground to manage a particular situation. In other cases it's better to "agree to disagree" and decide that one parent will handle a particular situation.

Good communication is crucial to a strong and effective partnership. Use the same strategies to improve communication between you and your spouse or parenting partner that you use with your child.

Having a positive, proactive stance toward managing your child's mood disorder and co-occurring symptoms will help your child, your family, and you. This chapter has reviewed some overarching principles to use as a guide. For more specific reading about general parenting strategies (e.g., communication with your child, discipline), see the Resources section at the back of this book.

9 | Coping Skills for Moody Children

We tend to think of kids as carefree, because they don't have to work for a living or handle the responsibilities of heading a family. But in truth it's not easy for kids to cope with all the challenges that arise in their social arena, at school, and at home. For children with mood disorders, the challenges are exponential. It's hard to find and maintain age-appropriate friendships and get along with kids in the neighborhood when you're struggling with irritability, decreased interest in activities, feelings of worthlessness, or low energy. And if mood symptoms have made you miss social events or have left you with a slightly unsavory social reputation, it can be hard to get back into the swing of things with your peers even after symptoms have abated. In school, behavioral problems caused by mood disorders can cause further social problems, as well as academic difficulties. Mood symptoms can make it hard to concentrate on class work and homework. Co-occurring conditions can put academic success even further out of reach. Home is the place that should be a haven, where everything should be easier, but even the safety of home can be disrupted when moodiness makes it hard for you to get along with family members and complete your chores, especially during acute phases of the illness.

Depression can make your son overly sensitive and hard to engage. Mania can make your daughter demanding and overly self-centered. Families often find that when they try to comfort or calm a child during a mood episode, their reassurances fall on deaf ears. At times negative behavior appears to occur "on purpose" and thus is more frustrating for family members to endure. Parents and siblings find it particularly trying when their child, brother, or sister wants (unsuccessfully) to be in control all the time. You and your family may feel like you're walking on eggshells to avoid unprovoked or violent outbursts, agitation, unpredictable or unreasonable behavior, and an apparent lack of caring for others.

Appropriate treatment, as described in Chapters 5 through 7, will help your child cope by lessening the effects of mood symptoms. But you can also help your child begin to build a set of skills and resources for managing her own symptoms. As symptom management improves, her ability to get along with friends, at school, and at home should improve as well.

As with all things, symptom management is different at each developmental level. Young children will rely much more heavily on adults for reminders and suggestions about using coping skills, whereas adolescents should be more self-sufficient. During acute phases of illness, increased assistance may be needed, regardless of your child's or teenager's age.

The "Tool Kit"

To fix a problem, you need tools that are specialized for the situation and the people involved. We like to think in terms of building a "tool kit" made up of different types of coping strategies and activities. Before fixing a problem, however, you and your child will need to think through what problems your child needs to fix.

Recall our discussion of problem solving in Chapter 8, as well as the "Naming the Enemy" exercise in Chapter 2. The first step is to define the problem. In what problem area does your child need assistance? For starters, turn to the symptoms you listed in the "Naming the Enemy" exercise. Is he irritable when he gets home from school? Does she have a very hard time settling down to do homework? Does he get sad over the weekend when he doesn't have the structure and activity of school? Is she irritable with friends during play dates? You may not be able to make these problems go away, but you can help your child develop strategies for managing them.

There are four basic types of activities that children can use to manage their own moods and other symptoms. Your child's tool kit should include some ideas from each category:

- Physical (e.g., running, jumping)
- Creative (e.g., drawing, building)
- Social (e.g., talking to a friend, petting the dog)
- Rest and relaxation (e.g., warm bath, herbal tea)

Even if your child is partial to one of these four categories (for example, you might have an artistic teen who loves to keep a journal, dance, and sing when she is feeling down), we recommend your child generate ideas from each category. This allows more flexibility in the heat of the moment when she has to pick a tool to use.

Your child's tool kit should be age appropriate. For a young child (from preschool through elementary school, depending on your child's level of maturity) the tool kit can be an actual box filled with real activities or symbols of those activities (e.g., the box might include a jump rope, some crayons and paper, the dog's favorite ball, and some granola bars). Some children enjoy decorating their box so that it looks special. For older children and adolescents, building the tool kit might involve making a list of choices within each area. (Figure 10 provides an example of activities that might be included in a child's tool kit.)

Kevin is ten, does well in school, and has several close friends. He gets frustrated easily, and his after-school irritability makes completing

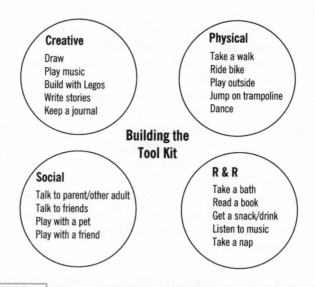

Creative
Draw
Play music
Build with Legos
Write stories
Keep a journal

Physical
Take a walk
Ride bike
Play outside
Jump on trampoline
Dance

Building the Tool Kit

Social
Talk to parent/other adult
Talk to friends
Play with a pet
Play with a friend

R & R
Take a bath
Read a book
Get a snack/drink
Listen to music
Take a nap

FIGURE 10 An example of activities that might be included in a child's tool kit.

homework difficult. It has also created some tension between Kevin and his eight-year-old sister, Abby. After a particularly trying afternoon, Kevin's mother, Melissa, sat down with him to build his tool kit. She asked Kevin to list things he enjoys in each area. Under "physical" he listed jumping on the trampoline, shooting baskets, and riding his bike. Under "creative" he listed building with Legos and playing the recorder. Under "social" he listed playing with his hamster, talking with his mom or dad, and playing with friends. Under "rest and relaxation" (R & R) he listed having a snack, getting a drink, and lying on his bed listening to music. Together they decided to keep several of Kevin's favorite CDs and his portable CD player in a box under his bed so that he would always be able to find them when he needed them. They posted the list on the back of Kevin's bedroom door, and he agreed to try something from his list when he got home from school. His mother agreed to give him time to relax before suggesting he start his homework.

Adam is six and wakes up in a grumpy funk most mornings even though he gets plenty of sleep (from 8:30 P.M. to 7:30 A.M.). His grumpy mood makes it very difficult for his mother, Kim, to get herself and Adam ready. She rarely gets to work on time after dropping Adam off at the sitter's, where he waits for the school bus. Kim helped Adam make a list of things he likes to do, such as dancing to music (physical), building with blocks and playing with action figures (creative), playing with their dog (social), and watching TV (R&R). To make these ideas more concrete, Kim and Adam decorated a box and labeled it "Tool Kit." They put his favorite CD, his blocks, some of his action figures, and a couple of dog toys in it. They decided that Kim would wake Adam and help him get started on a fun activity. She would then finish getting dressed and preparing his breakfast, which he would take to eat at the sitter's. Kim would then remind Adam to get dressed. If he had any extra time, Adam could watch TV until it was time to go. Starting his day with something fun really helped Adam's mood and eased their morning woes.

Adrian is a typical teen—she loves to listen to music, stay up late on-line with her friends, and would rather not have to get up early for school every morning. One thing (actually, more than one) sets Adrian apart from her peers, though. Adrian tried to kill herself last month. She's been out of the hospital, in which she spent six days and was diagnosed with depression, for weeks now, and she's been doing a pretty good job of remembering to take her medicine and going to therapy. Her school has a social worker, Mrs. Phillipi, in the building whom Adrian sees every Thursday during her lunch period.

Adrian's dad, Brian, is understandably concerned about how Adrian is doing. As a single dad, he feels like he's juggling as many balls as he can handle. Maintaining some semblance of a routine for his two younger boys while Adrian was in the hospital nearly wore him out. However, he's worried that Adrian might be heading back into trouble. She's staying up late, way past the time he's able to manage to stay up to keep an eye on her, and she's already missed a day of school this week because she couldn't wake up on time. Brian called Mrs. Phillipi to get some advice. She shared his concern that Adrian is staying up too late, as that would likely lead to Adrian missing school the next day, which could start a downward spiral—missing school would lead to an unsupervised day at home, which neither of them thought was a good idea. Mrs. Phillipi suggested that Brian ask Adrian to show him her tool kit, which they worked on together in therapy this past Thursday.

That night after dinner, Brian told Adrian about his call to Mrs. Phillipi and shared his concern with Adrian that she was staying up past midnight every night. Adrian told her dad he didn't need to worry but seemed relieved that he was taking an interest in her struggles. After her two younger brothers went to bed, she dug the tool kit out of her backpack. On a piece of paper, Mrs. Phillipi had drawn four ovals, and Adrian had written in ideas to use when she was feeling really sad or lonely. Adrian reviewed the four ovals to pick ideas that would help her feel calm and peaceful as she was getting ready for bed, as that is the time that negative, anxious, and sad thoughts tend to flood her mind. She decided that the "physical" category would get her too wound up, rather than putting her into a mellow mood—she would save those ideas for the afternoons when she came home from school. Likewise, the "creative" category wasn't appropriate—Adrian loves to sing, but she can't do that late at night after her brothers are in bed. Adrian was already using ideas from the "social" category—instant messaging and talking on the phone to her friends. Despite moaning and groaning, Adrian agreed to stop doing that by 11:00 P.M. so that she could use the next half-hour to quietly unwind and prepare herself for bed. That left the "R & R" category—Adrian chose the "hot washcloth" idea from her list. After getting all ready for bed, Adrian would get a steaming hot washcloth ready, then lie in bed with it on her face. This had a way of relaxing all the muscles in her face and neck, where Adrian's tension tends to accumulate. When she was done with it, she'd dry her face with a towel she had waiting, then drop them both by the side of her bed as she fell asleep.

Although Brian would have preferred that Adrian pick 10:30 or 11:00

P.M. as her bedtime, 11:30 P.M. was a reasonable compromise, because she had been going to bed around 1:00 each morning. They agreed to monitor this arrangement for a week. If Adrian still was struggling in the morning one week later, they would move her bedtime back to 11:15 P.M.

Using a tool kit, whether actual or figurative, is a good practical way to approach symptom management. In addition, the tool kit reinforces our favorite motto: It's not your fault, but it's your challenge (and you need the right tools to manage it)!

Divide and Conquer (Coping with Depression)

Depression can lead a child or teen to feel immobilized or overwhelmed. What seems to be a simple homework assignment to the parent can seem unmanageable to the child. Getting dressed in the morning can become a monstrous task. One way to help depressed children manage is to teach them to "divide and conquer" by breaking tasks into manageable chunks.

Kayla is twelve and has recently started therapy to help with her depressed feelings and worrying. Although she is a bright and capable student, she is frequently overwhelmed by her homework assignments. She becomes tearful and immobilized. Her father is her best ally at these times. In a calm and matter-of-fact manner, he helps her make a list of her assignments and break them into smaller chunks. He also reassures her that if she can't complete everything, he'll write a note to her teacher. He has yet to write that note.

Putting on the Brakes (Managing Mania)

During manic and hypomanic episodes, energy and motivation run high. You may notice that your son or daughter is starting more activities than usual. This may be a nuisance or may create significant problems down the line.

Griffin is fourteen and in high school. At the beginning of a hypomanic episode, he was feeling on top of the world and began getting involved in multiple activities. He joined a number of activities, including signing up for the stage crew for the school play, joining the decorations committee for the homecoming dance, and trying out for the cross-country team. His mother noticed that he was getting overextended and tried to talk about it with him. He immediately got defensive and stormed off to his room. Feeling defeated, his mother left him alone. A week later, Griffin's energy level and mood began to drop. He became more irritable and sad and had just enough energy to get through school and finish his homework. He quickly became overwhelmed by all of his commitments.

Griffin's situation illustrates what can happen during a period of hypomania or mania. With an elevated mood and high energy, he joined several activities. While Griffin's mood stayed up, he was able to keep up the pace. As his mood dropped into depression, he was no longer able to. An added risk is that being overcommitted can lead teens to stay up late and put themselves at further risk for more severe mood symptoms (sleep deprivation can sometimes lead to manic episodes or can lead to daytime napping followed by nighttime insomnia).

A useful concept for managing mania is "putting on the brakes." As manic symptoms develop, it is important to maintain a normal level of activity so that, when mania subsides, there are no significant repercussions that may increase depressed feelings. Teenagers usually need to experience a "crash and burn" a time or two before they can internalize the need for limiting activities as they are going into a hypomanic state.

Don't Give Away the Answer

A key ingredient for success here is that parents not give the solution to their teenager or child. Rather, they can use Socratic questioning to help their teenager find his own solution, asking a series of questions to help the child arrive at a particular conclusion, rather than telling him the solution.

Elizabeth was tired of listening to her seventeen-year-old daughter, Julia, complain about her teachers, her peers, her boss at work, and her thirteen-year-old brother. Julia had been diagnosed with dysthymic disorder (DD) two months earlier. She had begun to see a therapist and started taking Lexapro, an antidepressant. Julia was making some progress. She seemed to have more energy, perhaps because she was falling asleep more quickly at night. However, from her point of view, her cup was still half empty. When Julia started her Saturday morning by complaining about what a moron her boss was, Elizabeth snapped. She started screaming at Julia that if she would just stop being so negative, maybe her life wouldn't be so miserable. Julia gave her mother a withering look, said, "Maybe you're the one who ought to be in therapy, not me!" and waltzed off.

Elizabeth pondered their horrible morning for the rest of the day. She was convinced that it was Julia who had the biggest problem, but she did feel at her wit's end in terms of how to help her. When Julia came home from work that evening, Elizabeth approached her, saying that Julia had a point. Elizabeth really could use some time with Julia's therapist, so perhaps she could spend part of Julia's next session to get her questions answered. Julia said that would be fine with her.

Next Tuesday, Elizabeth drove Julia to her appointment (Julia usually drove herself there). She asked Julia's social worker, Kaye, if she could use part of the session for her questions. Kaye readily agreed. Elizabeth confessed about the miserable interchange they had the previous Saturday. Kaye helped Elizabeth label the tension she has felt about Julia, in particular how worried Elizabeth is about how Julia will do in the future, especially after she graduates from high school. Kaye explained how physical symptoms of depression usually improve first. (Julia's sleep had improved and her fatigue had decreased.) Mood and thought patterns tend to improve at a slower pace. Kaye acknowledged that Julia had very entrenched negative thoughts, seemingly about everyone and everything. Kaye coached Elizabeth in Socratic questioning. Rather than giving Julia "the answer" (in this case, "stop looking at life in such a negative way"), Elizabeth could best help Julia by getting her to come to this realization on her own. Using Saturday as an example, Kaye led Elizabeth through a way in which she could manage these negative moments in the future.

JULIA: My boss is such a moron!

ELIZABETH: Why do you say that?

JULIA: You wouldn't believe what he did Thursday night as we were closing!

ELIZABETH: Really, what was that?

JULIA: He forgot to take the money out of the cash register! How dumb can that be?

ELIZABETH: Wow, I wonder if he was preoccupied—you know, thinking about something else at the same time. Remember when that happened to you when you were supposed to go to your dental appointment?

JULIA: Oh yeah, boy, was that stupid of me! I totally forgot and drove to work instead, and I wasn't even scheduled to be there!

ELIZABETH: And remember what you did after that, to help yourself stay more organized?

JULIA: Yeah, I started putting sticky notes in the car to remind myself when I had to go different places.

ELIZABETH: Makes me wonder—think Rick, your boss, might need sticky notes, too?

JULIA: Yeah, maybe he could put one on the cash register that says "Don't forget to empty me!" (*Laughs.*)

ELIZABETH: (*Hugs Julia.*) It's nice to hear you laughing again, honey. I've really missed that sound in our house.

Choose the Right Man/Woman for the Job

It's also advisable for parents to decide who can best "keep their cool" over any particular issue. Different topics tend to hit the "hot button" for different parents. For example, one parent might do best with a discussion over choices of friends, whereas the other parent might be more effective in a conversation about schoolwork.

When Griffin started heading into a "high," his father, Tom (who is particularly good at staying calm when problem solving is needed), sat down to have a conversation with Griffin. Tom asked how Griffin had been doing lately, how connected he was feeling to the other kids in his new, large high school, what activities he was finding the most enjoyable, and whether he ever felt overwhelmed by all the choices of activities and number of classes he was taking. Through a series of questions, Tom was able to lead Griffin into identifying how he can get too caught up in too many commitments. Tom gently pursued his questioning until Griffin developed his own plan to monitor the number of activities he would allow himself to begin. Griffin decided on a plan to add no more than one new activity at a time until he became acclimated to that level of commitment in his schedule. Tom then asked Griffin if they could go out for breakfast one Saturday morning a month to talk about how his busy freshman year was going. Griffin thought that was a great idea.

Making a Sleep Plan

Maintaining a good sleep schedule is important for all children. For children and adolescents with mood disorders, it's crucial. Insufficient sleep contributes to more depression, and more depression can lead to poorer sleep—and thus a vicious cycle ensues. Additionally, poor sleep habits can precipitate manic episodes. So you need a sleep plan. For children, the responsibility for managing sleep falls mainly on parents. This means establishing and maintaining a reasonable bedtime, sticking with a routine, and keeping a consistent waking time. On weekends and vacations, the ideal is not to let the sleep routine change by more than one hour (e.g., if regular bedtime is 8:30 P.M., weekend bedtimes should be no later than 9:30 P.M.).

This gets more difficult as children grow into teenagers who keep a different set of hours. We encourage you to talk over and solve this problem with your teenager. However, keep in mind that teens need to be more self-reliant in developing and maintaining a sleep plan. They are likely to resist too much parental involvement, so sleep may be a good topic for your teen to discuss with his therapist. Teenagers tend to be chronically sleep deprived. A common practice is to try to catch up on the weekends. This may be tolerable for teens without mood disorders, but it can create significant problems for teens with depression and bipolar disorder.

Prevention Is the Best Medicine

In Chapter 5 we talked about separating "can't" behavior from "won't" behavior. It is certainly true that once your child reaches the "can't" stage, your goal will need to shift to deescalating his mood. However, there are steps you and your child can take before he gets to that point. The tool kit we introduced earlier in this chapter provides a way for your child to engage actively in disaster prevention. The better he becomes at using his tool kit, the less likely you are to have those horrific battles or miserable moments. Additionally, you and your child can engage in what behavior therapists do—analyzing your ABCs to see what low points you can prevent.

ABC stands for *antecedents, behaviors,* and *consequences*. Antecedents are what precedes the behavior you want to avoid: your miserably depressed thirteen-year-old telling you life isn't worth living while he is holed up in his darkened bedroom; your seven-year-old raging beyond control while destroying the family room; or your sixteen-year-old flying higher than a kite as she exits the front door in a garish outfit. What families have told us over time, which research literature supports, is that certain triggers can contribute to making matters much, much worse. After you read through the following list, you might feel that no one could be at their best under such conditions. That is true, but the point we want to make is that children and teenagers with mood disorders often do *tremendously* worse under these conditions.

Triggers to Avoid

- *Heat.* Watch those summer months (and sweltering spring and fall classrooms) carefully. Make sure your child gets cooled off, or, in situations in which heat can't be avoided, keep fluid intake sufficient to prevent dehydration.

- *Hunger.* Anticipate the need for snacks. If your child is taking medication that contributes to weight gain, be prepared with high-nutrition, high-fiber, low-calorie snacks. Avoid soft drinks and fruit drinks; they are filled with empty calories.

- *Fatigue.* Many tired children will deny that fatigue is contributing to their lousy mood. Reread the section on sleep earlier in this chapter.

- *Overstimulation.* Too much commotion (e.g., visitors in the home, extended travel over a holiday) can wear down your child's patience (and yours as well). Pace your family's activities in a way that all can be successful.

- *Understimulation.* Particularly for depressed children, not having enough to do can contribute to their curling up into a withdrawn ball or lashing out at "boring" siblings. Working with your child and her therapist on what we refer to as *activity scheduling* (ensuring that pleasurable activities are built into her day-to-day routine) can stave off some of these difficulties.

After you've become familiar with watching for antecedents—those situations that repeatedly precede a bad spell—also begin to watch for the consequences of these behaviors. Do you find that you give in after your child has a mood meltdown or appears to be on the verge of having one? If so, is your child being inadvertently rewarded for these behaviors?

Eight-year-old Joey has had bipolar disorder essentially his entire life. He was diagnosed at age five. Although treatment has helped, there are times when he becomes manically fixated on a seemingly silly or impractical desire. For example, after flipping through a toy catalog one evening, Joey insisted that his mother drive him to the nearest toy store to purchase a particular action figure. Despite her best reasoning, he could not be dissuaded from his quest. The problem was that Joey's dad worked evenings, and his mother couldn't leave Joey's five-year-old sister Emily home alone while they made the trek to the toy store. So Mom redressed Emily from her pajamas into play clothes, and off they went. Much to his mother's ire, Joey played with his new action figure toy for about ten minutes after they got home, then tossed it into the large bin with all his other action figures, not to play with it again for days.

At their next therapy appointment, Joey's counselor was able to help his mom understand the difference between avoiding triggers (e.g., making sure Joey has a variety of toys available with which he can play, alone or with others) and being manipulated out of fear that a rage will ensue.

Getting the Signal

Softball and baseball teams often use elaborate signals to tell players when to run, steal a base, or bunt. All the players and coaches learn these signals and agree to use them. You may find a similar system to be useful with your child. Children are often embarrassed when their parents try to help out by pulling them out of situations. Using simple signals can provide a private way for parents to help their children self-regulate and avoid negative situations. For example, when Sean starts to get overexcited, his mother calls him into the house to help her with something. The break gives Sean a chance to calm down and is done in a way that doesn't embarrass him. Nonverbal cues can also be used if the child is able to pick up on them. Prior to beginning to use the signals, parents and children should agree on the signals and how and when they will be used.

Relapse Prevention

Let's suppose you and your child have been working hard—learning about her mood disorder, initiating treatment, and following through with therapy. Now you're rewarded with your child's improvement. Your therapist has told you to call her on an as-needed basis, because your son is doing so well. Your psychiatrist recommended cutting down visits to every six months unless problems arise. What should you do? You cannot and should not try to become your child's therapist. However, you are the one who sees your child every day. You have relative control over his schedule. You are best equipped to help your child avoid events or situations that might precipitate a relapse. Review what we've discussed in this chapter so far regarding how your child can help himself. If you feel stuck, call your child's therapist for an appointment. Being prepared to spot troublesome patterns early in their development can help you and your child nip it in the bud.

We've shared some coping strategies you can use to help your child or teen manage the day-to-day struggles that come with mood disorders. By building a tool kit, then using strategies such as divide and conquer, putting on the brakes, working on communication, dividing up

---

TIPS FOR PARENTS: WHAT SHOULD YOU AVOID?

- Reassuring your child too rapidly (e.g., "Everything's fine!").
- Reinterpreting your child's perceptions (e.g., "It's not as bad as you think—I'm sure you have friends at school").
- Taking comments literally or personally. If your child says "I hate you!" or "You're the worst parent I could ever have had!" in the midst of a rage episode, remind yourself that this is the mood disorder, not your child, talking.
- Attempting to be constantly available and positive. As much as you love your child, you need breaks, and you are human, too!
- Feeling guilty for not meeting your child's every need. Guilt is rarely helpful. Besides, you have needs, too, as do your other family members.
- Allowing the disorder to take over family life (e.g., avoiding family outings for fear of an incident occurring).
- Making big decisions (e.g., about custody, job changes, divorce) during an episode. These decisions may need to be made, but you need to make them with a clear head.

tasks, and developing healthy sleep patterns and signals to use with each other, you and your child can learn to manage the mood disorder rather than letting it manage you.

Keep in mind that one of the most important coping strategies is to seek appropriate help. Make sure you have adequate therapy and medication management. Although the techniques described in this chapter may be very helpful, they tend to work best with children or teenagers who are also utilizing other forms of treatment. If you and your child try these techniques without the proper amount of backup, you may become demoralized. Remember, use the communication and problem-solving strategies we discussed in Chapter 8 to decide what other help you may or may not need to manage your child's mood symptoms.

10 Mood Disorders in the School Setting

WHAT YOU NEED TO KNOW TO HELP YOUR CHILD COPE

Kids spend about half of their waking hours at school, so helping your child or teenager cope at school is important. Mood disorders can cause three types of problems for your child at school: problems caused by the core symptoms themselves (e.g., impaired concentration), problems caused by secondary factors (e.g., peer problems), and problems caused by the treatment (e.g., medication side effects or inconveniences related to treatment, such as needing to take medications at lunch time or regularly missing classes to attend therapy appointments). Additionally, many children and teens with mood disorders also have co-occurring learning disabilities, as we discussed in Chapter 4. These learning disabilities will require standard forms of intervention (see the Resources section for some educational suggestions), and educational staff should be aware of the additional levels of impaired concentration, reduced motivation, and so forth that the added mood disorder creates.

Problems Caused by Core Symptoms

Many symptoms of depression and mania make functioning in school very difficult.

Mood Changes

Extreme moods, whether sad, excessively happy, or angry, are particularly difficult for children and adolescents to manage at school.

Brandon was determined to make it through a full school day. He got to school on time (which was a monumental effort for him). Halfway through his favorite class (American history), he was overwhelmed by sadness. He lost track of what his teacher was saying about the Revolutionary War as he struggled to fight back tears.

Marla's mother sent her to school reluctantly. Marla had been going nonstop since she woke up at 5:00 A.M. Marla was *very* happy. *Too* happy. Marla was typically well behaved at school. Today, however, she was really struggling. Everything her teacher said seemed funny to her, and she kept laughing when no one else in the class was laughing. When she started giggling uncontrollably during math, Mrs. Dee suggested that Marla go to the office to calm down for a little while. Marla was appalled. She had never gotten in trouble at school before.

Dante is very irritable. He scowls at teachers, students, and anyone else who crosses his path. Today a classmate cut ahead of him in the lunch line. Something inside Dante exploded, and he threw his lunch tray at the boy, who jumped away to avoid being hit. Dante's tray ended up knocking over some glass containers at the end of the lunch line. Broken glass spewed all over the cafeteria floor. Dante just stared stone-faced at the mess he had created. The principal called Dante into her office and placed him in the in-school suspension room for the rest of the day.

As you can imagine, intense moods can significantly disrupt the learning experience of a child or teenager with a mood disorder.

Loss of Interest

One of the core symptoms of depression is loss of interest in activities. For many children and adolescents with depression, this means a loss of interest in school and schoolwork.

Although Brandon still wanted to do well in school, he just couldn't muster the energy or interest to write his history paper. Two months ago, before his depression really took hold, Brandon had chosen the topic for his paper, and he had been excited to learn about patterns of immigration to the United States. Now Brandon could hardly fathom the thought of going to the library, let alone reading the books and writing the paper.

Loss of interest in school can create a vicious cycle. Not completing work results in lower grades, and for many, lower grades can lead to a lowered self-opinion.

Fatigue

Depression can also lead to fatigue. School participation can be very difficult when you can barely keep your head up and you have no energy.

Brandon dragged himself out of bed, with his mother encouraging him every step of the way. Several times he gave up and got back in bed. He finally made it to school. His first class, English, was a good one, but it didn't matter. As soon as he was seated, Brandon was fighting sleep. About fifteen minutes into class he was embarrassed to realize that his teacher was tapping him on the shoulder because he had fallen asleep. His sympathetic teacher wrote him a note and sent him to the nurse's office.

Concentration

Difficulty concentrating can be particularly frustrating for children and adolescents who typically excel academically but find themselves unable to stay focused and think clearly because of their mood disorders.

Brandon sat down one evening in an attempt to complete his English class reading assignment. After sitting at his desk for twenty minutes and reading only one paragraph, Brandon burst into tears and put his head down on his arms. His mother heard him crying and came to see what was wrong. Through his tears Brandon told her that he couldn't concentrate well enough even to read a novel.

Agitation and Retardation

In addition to fatigue and general slowing, depression can sometimes result in psychomotor agitation or retardation. Psychomotor agitation can cause an individual to feel driven to move (e.g., pace, tap a foot) and can result in significant problems in the classroom.

Kayla is a good student who has never had behavioral problems at school. Recently, though, she has been struggling with being sad and having to force herself to stay focused on her work. Kayla was surprised when the boy next to her hissed "Stop it!" at her while they were working on a math assignment. She realized that she had been tapping her foot nonstop. Kayla tried to quit, but the more she tried, the more she just felt like she needed to move. Kayla's mother had also commented on her tapping and fidgeting over the previous few days.

Depression can also cause psychomotor retardation, which makes a person appear to be in "slow motion."

Marcus, a high school junior, was late to his fifth-period math class every day for two weeks. Finally his teacher said—in front of the whole class—that she needed to have a conference with him after class. When she asked him what was going on, Marcus just shook his head. He hadn't been doing anything in particular that made him late; he just couldn't make his legs go any faster.

It's normal for people to have particular times of day when they are most efficient or energetic (e.g., most of us would describe ourselves as either early birds or night owls). But with mood disorders, changes in energy level can be more dramatic, with periods of hyperactivity that can make seated work difficult and/or periods of lethargy that make timely completion of any activity a struggle.

Four-year-old Ben has just been diagnosed with bipolar disorder and now is in the process of being stabilized on medications. In the meantime, Ben's preschool teachers have been working closely with his parents. Ben's teachers have noted that Ben tends to have periods of extremely high activity during the first part of the morning and to be less active and more focused later in the morning. To better accommodate Ben, his teachers agreed to move group circle time to 11:00 A.M. instead of 9:00 A.M. so that Ben can gain more from the experience. Ben's teachers have also arranged for Ben to go straight to the playground (when weather permits) upon his arrival to burn off a little energy.

Poor Judgment

Mania and hypomania can frequently result in questionable decision making. Poor judgment can lead to dangerous or embarrassing activities, such as making sexual comments, being excessively daring, or bragging about perceived abilities.

Marla enjoyed singing, and one day she was sure that she had the best voice in her class. During chorus Marla sang as loud as she could. Twice the chorus teacher asked her to sing more softly. Marla was irritated by the teacher's obvious lack of appreciation for her talent and proceeded to sing even louder. At one point Marla's best friend whispered to her that she was singing too loud. Marla shot her a withering look and continued to sing as loud as she could.

Racing Thoughts

Mania and hypomania often bring rapid or racing thoughts, which can make it very difficult to focus on what is going on around you. Listening to and processing school lessons will not go smoothly.

Marla had so many ideas about what to do after school—her thoughts were swirling around and around in her head. Her efforts to pay attention to the math paper that was sitting on her desk in front of her were futile. Despite Marla's teacher's reminders that she had to finish the paper or she would have to do it as extra homework, Marla had barely started the first problem before the period ended.

Pressured Speech

Mania and hypomania also frequently bring pressured speech or the sensation that words just can't get out fast enough. Marla loved reading. She especially loved class discussions about the books they read as a class. When the teacher started asking questions about their current book, Marla eagerly raised her hand. The teacher called on her, and Marla started talking a mile a minute. Marla neglected to answer the teacher's question but talked on and on about the book. Finally, the teacher had to say Marla's name loudly to get her attention and to get her to stop talking.

Problems Caused by Secondary Factors

Peer Problems

Peer problems are among the most devastating and long-lasting consequences of mood disorders. Depression can lead to social withdrawal, and, as peer networks can be fragile, turning down a few invitations from a child to play can result in no further invitations from that person. As children learn social skills by interacting with others, lost opportunities to play are lost opportunities to learn. Failure to learn age-appropriate social skills can cause a child to fall further and further behind socially and to be included less often by her peer group.

Sarah is eight and has been diagnosed with dysthymic disorder. She had been unhappy for so long that, prior to treatment (she is now on an antidepressant and working with a therapist), she didn't know what a happy mood was like. Sarah was often withdrawn at recess and rejected most opportunities to play with other girls in her class. With treatment, Sarah was happier. She became interested in playing with her peers. Although the other children in her class were mostly nice, they had well-developed friendships and didn't think to include Sarah in their games. This resulted in Sarah's feeling lonely and unsure about how to become part of the group. With her therapist, Sarah came up with some ideas to initiate contact. She began saying "hi" to several girls in her class each morning. She also invited one of the quieter girls over to her house to play. Gradually, Sarah began to be included in group projects during the school day, as well as in games at recess.

In addition to the problems caused by social withdrawal, excessive peer conflict can be a major impediment for children with mood disorders.

Lauren is nine years old and bossy. At the height of her mood symptoms, her classmates avoided her: They were never sure when she would explode at them. Now that she is taking an effective combination of medications, she is less explosive but still bossy. Lauren has frequent arguments with peers and at times has started physical fights. It's getting hard for Lauren to find kids who will play with her because of her reputation for being a bossy, know-it-all bully.

The quality, as well as quantity, of friendships can be affected by mood disorders. Because "misery loves company," mood-impaired children and teens often gravitate toward others with similar problems. Although having friends who understand what you are going through is helpful, having a social network composed exclusively of others with impairing conditions can also be problematic. Helping your child make some social contacts based on similar hobbies or interests (e.g., marching band, church youth group) can help prevent an "exclusive club" from forming.

Other Secondary Problems

Being socially isolated as a result of mood symptoms can create many problems. If a child spends the whole morning worrying about what child to play with at recess, he will not be focusing on his teacher's lessons. Another child might act out to avoid socially stressful times of day—being sent to the office or given a detention may seem like a better deal than facing the "recess gauntlet." The possible problems that can arise are as varied as the children with mood disorders themselves. As your child's advocate, be aware of what problems your child is having and be creative along with school staff in your attempts to understand and solve them.

Problems Caused by Treatment

Medication Side Effects

Medication side effects can range from an easily accommodated nuisance to a cause of significant interference with school functioning. Some side effects are extremely embarrassing (for example, lithium can lead to bladder accidents), and some are uncomfortable (for example, feeling very thirsty or having a dry mouth). Some medications cause sedation that can further interfere with school. Reread Chapter 6, especially the section on side-effect management, to think through ways to manage these difficulties at school.

Other Problems Caused by Treatment

Although treatment providers strive to cause as little interference as possible, at times treatment itself can create some problems. For example, although a simple medication regimen is often preferable, some children need a dose of medication during the school day. This means that the school has to store and administer medication on a daily basis and that school personnel and the child have to remember when the medication should be taken. For schools with a full-time nurse (which is not common), this is easier. In other cases, medication is dispensed by principals, teachers, or even secretaries. In addition, children often find leaving class to go take medication embarrassing. Finally, needing to leave school at the same time every week or two weeks for therapy appointments can cause a student already struggling to stay on top of her homework to fall even further behind. Some clinicians offer evening and weekend hours, but many do not. It will be important to work out plans with your child's school to ensure that these problems can be addressed adequately. In the following pages we give you ideas about working effectively with your child's school to accomplish these goals.

What Can I Do?

Accommodating a child with a mood disorder at school can be as simple as arranging minor changes with your child's teacher (e.g., unlimited access to the bathroom) or as complicated as developing an individualized education plan (IEP) with multiple behavioral and academic goals and a range of service providers. The cost of educational interventions range from none to high. No-cost and low-cost interventions require cooperation and flexibility, whereas moderate-cost and high-cost interventions require financial resources.

To help you determine what is best for your child, we first provide you with some overarching principles to keep in mind as you work with your child's school. Second, we summarize key points about special education law and lingo, the range of available services, and how to access services. Third, we provide some examples of how the educational needs of children and adolescents with mood disorders might be met. Finally, because interacting effectively with schools when addressing the needs of a mood-disordered child can be a complex matter, we've included additional resources concerning how to work effectively with schools and how to devise classroom and curriculum modifications for your child in the Resources section.

A Collaborative, Realistic Approach

Although you might need to push hard to get the services your child needs, keep in mind that you need to collaborate with your child's school to develop your child's educational team. As long as you live in your current school district, you will be working with the same school personnel (or their colleagues, if your child transfers schools or moves up from middle school to high school).

Your child's teacher(s), principal, guidance counselor, and other school employees make up your child's educational team. Part of your job is to establish collaborative relationships with members of the team. Your team may be small (i.e., you, your child, and your child's teacher) or extensive (i.e., you and your spouse, your child's other biological parent and his or her spouse, your child, your child's mainstream teacher and special education teacher, your child's guidance counselor and principal, and your child's speech and language therapist). Regardless of your team's size, it is important to work together to create the best possible educational program given your child's needs and the available resources.

Although you should always ask for everything your child needs, recognize that the school is limited by its available resources. It would be wonderful if all schools could provide for every child's every need. Unfortunately, resources are much more limited than we would like. So look for alternatives. If your home school has a specialized behavioral classroom[1] that tends to serve only kids who are more severely impaired than your child, does one of the other schools in the district have a similar resource room? Do you know anything about surrounding districts? Is moving feasible? Is it a good option?

> ### TIPS FOR PARENTS: DOS AND DON'TS FOR WORKING WITH YOUR CHILD'S EDUCATIONAL TEAM
>
> *DO:*
> 1. Explore all possibilities.
> 2. Ask for all services that you think are relevant.
> 3. Do your homework and be well educated about what your child needs and the resources previously made available in your district (and elsewhere) for children with similar needs.
> 4. Be collaborative. Make suggestions and be receptive to other suggestions.
> 5. Know your rights and your child's rights.
>
> *DON'T:*
> 1. Be demanding.
> 2. Refuse to listen to alternatives.
> 3. Make threats.

Understanding the Law

Two different federal laws dictate how educational services are managed. Having an understanding of the mechanics of school programming will help you as a parent know what to ask for in a meeting.

THE INDIVIDUALS WITH DISABILITIES EDUCATION ACT (IDEA)

IDEA is a 1997 federal law (revision of 1973 law) guaranteeing a "free and appropriate education" (FAPE) in the "least restrictive environment" (LRE) along with appropriate "related services." The law requires

---

[1]The terms and abbreviations used to describe special education services vary from state to state and even district to district. Your state's board of education should be able to provide a pamphlet that explains terminology and abbreviations. See the Resource section for suggestions about how to contact your state's board of education.

a multifactored evaluation (MFE) to determine eligibility for children with potential disabilities.

SECTION 504 OF THE 1973 REHABILITATION ACT

This is a civil rights law prohibiting discrimination against anyone with a disability. Section 504 provides the right to participate in programs and activities that receive federal financial assistance (i.e., public schools). This law is useful if your child's condition requires accommodations but she does not qualify under IDEA. Table 4 describes the differences between IDEA and Section 504.

KNOW THE LINGO!

The only place where you will encounter more abbreviations than on Wall Street is at your local school. You need an MFE to get an IEP that specifies your FAPE in the LRE! Sound like gibberish? See Table 5 for definitions of common terms and abbreviations.

SPECIAL EDUCATION SERVICES

For some children, adjustments and plans for accommodation are not enough to allow success in a regular classroom. For these children, special education services are necessary. These services can range from those provided within the regular classroom (inclusion), to the child

TABLE 4	IDEA versus 504	
Mechanism	Individuals with Disabilities Education Act (IDEA)	Section 504 of the Rehabilitation Act
Eligibility	Must meet 1 of 13 qualifying categories	Eligible if handicapping condition is present
Requirements	Written IEP based on an MFE	An agreed-upon 504 plan
Advantages	Federal money to the district, more extensive modifications/ services	Expedient, often more flexible
Disadvantages	Requires more paperwork, time to complete, testing	No additional money to the district, often not adhered to as strictly or consistently

| TABLE 5 | Definitions of Common Educational Terms and Abbreviations |

Abbreviation or term	Name	Definition
FAPE	Free and appropriate education	School districts must provide all eligible students with special education and related services allowing personalized instruction and sufficient support services necessary to permit the child to benefit educationally at the public's expense.
MFE	Multifactored evaluation	Evaluation completed by the school (by a multidisciplinary team) to determine eligibility for special services. Ensures that no single procedure is the sole criterion for determining a child's eligibility for services.
IEE	Independent educational evaluation	Every parent has a right to obtain an IEE at the expense of the school if they are dissatisfied with the multifactored evaluation and if they have followed specific procedural requirements of the law.
FBA	Functional behavioral assessment	An evaluation, usually conducted by a school psychologist, to identify triggers that precede losses of control or other significant behavioral problems.
IEP	Individualized education program	Specific plan devised by school personnel with parent participation and approval. Establishes child's educational goals and how they will be met.
LRE	Least restrictive environment	Placement that provides needed educational services while maintaining maximum participation in regular education services with typical peers.
Due process	Due process	Parental right to approve or disapprove of plans proposed by the school or district special services team and to engage a review process if the plan does not meet approval.
OHI	Other health impaired	A classification for children whose health problems (e.g., bipolar disorder, depression) adversely affect school performance and prevent the children's needs from being met entirely by regular education services.
SLD	Specific learning disability	Achievement in particular academic areas (e.g., reading, math) are below expected levels based on tested ability level.
Mainstreaming	Mainstreaming	Children who have been placed in a self-contained classroom rejoin their regular class for particular classes or time periods. Sometimes used as an incentive for children with behavioral challenges or as a transition from a self-contained classroom back to a regular classroom.

(continued)

Abbreviation or Term	Name	Definition
Inclusion	Inclusion	All special education services are provided within the context of the regular classroom with typical peers. A special education teacher coordinates services, oversees implementation of the IEP, and consults with the classroom teacher.
SBH	Severe behavioral handicap	Term used to describe children who have significant behavioral dysregulation.
SED	Severe emotional disturbance	Term used to describe children who have significant emotional needs.

spending some time in a resource room designed to support children with emotional and behavioral needs, to placement in a self-contained classroom.

Regular Classroom plus Support from a Resource Room or Special Education Teacher. This is a highly flexible arrangement. Resource-room support for a child in a regular classroom placement can be set up in a variety of ways. Depending on the child's needs, he could spend either most of the day or no time in the resource room. The resource room is meant to serve as a support for the child during difficult times. A child who tends to have particular behavioral problems during math class might go to the resource room each day at that time. Alternatively, a child who does well most of the time but has periods of being very irritable might go to the resource room when he needs a quiet place to work and an opportunity to settle himself down. Typically, resource rooms are staffed by a special education teacher and an aide. Although not actually designed to act in that way, the SBH or SED resource room is sometimes used as a self-contained classroom. For some children, the resource room is used to facilitate the transition from a self-contained class back to a regular class. In some cases, a child would stay in the regular classroom, and a special education teacher would join the regular class for parts of the day to provide support.

Self-Contained Classroom. Self-contained classrooms vary from district to district and state to state. These classrooms are typically staffed by at least one special education teacher and at least one aide.

The student–teacher ratio is significantly smaller than in the regular classroom.

Inclusion Programs. Special education services are handled differently in each state and district. Some schools use inclusion as their primary mode of serving children with special needs. A child with significant needs might require a one-on-one aide to function successfully in the regular classroom. Good inclusion programs have a special education teacher who works closely with the regular teacher and the child. Academic and behavioral goals and plans for how to meet those goals should be specified in the IEP. As with self-contained classrooms, a well-qualified and supported staff with adequate resources is probably more important than the educational philosophy being used.

Therapeutic Day School. Children often are recommended for therapeutic schools when they have been unable to function in regular schools. Unlike regular schools that have the primary goal of teaching academic subjects, therapeutic schools have dual goals. They focus both on academics and on social and emotional functioning. Therapy groups, as well as behavioral programs, are likely to be part of the school day.

A Hospital's Day Treatment Program. Child and adolescent inpatient units often have a day treatment program available. During the day, children attend school, participate in therapeutic activities, and then return home for the evening. Participation in a day treatment program is typically brief and serves as a transition from hospital to return to home or school.

Residential Treatment Center. When children are unable to function at school and at home, sometimes a residential treatment center is needed. Residential programs have schools, along with the full range of therapeutic services.

Therapeutic Boarding Schools. Usually designed for adolescents and older children, therapeutic boarding schools may have a military or college preparation focus. These programs tend to provide a good education along with therapeutic services, but they tend to be expensive and usually are not covered by insurance.

In addition to knowing school programming options, it is important to know who the various personnel at school are.

Who's Who?: Know the Educational Team Players

TEACHERS

The frontline players on the educational team are teachers. At the elementary school level, children will typically have only one or possibly two classroom teachers. At the middle and high school levels, your adolescent is likely to have several teachers and will probably move from classroom to classroom to meet those teachers. In many cases this will make your job more challenging; you will have to work harder to figure out with whom to speak when things aren't going as expected. Special education teachers may serve a consulting role (i.e., providing support for classroom teachers; meeting with children with special needs in the regular classroom or in the resource room on an as-needed basis), or they may run a self-contained classroom. Teachers will vary in their level of understanding of mental health issues. Offer to provide reading material. Although most teachers are willing to learn, their training quite likely did not include detailed information about childhood mood disorders.

GUIDANCE COUNSELORS

The availability of guidance counselors will vary from district to district and age to age. Some elementary schools will not have guidance counselors or will have one guidance counselor who serves several schools. Find out if your child's school has a guidance counselor and, if so, how much time he or she is available. Guidance counselors can serve in many different roles depending on the school, on their training, and on their responsibilities. Some possibilities include holding regular or as-needed one-on-one meetings with children who are struggling socially or emotionally, running social skills groups during school hours, providing alternative activities during stressful unstructured times (many children with mood disorders struggle socially and find recess and lunchtime to be particularly difficult), running whole-class programs on topics such as stress management, and consulting with classroom teachers. If your school has a guidance counselor available, he or she may be willing and able to serve a range of functions. The bottom line is, *ask or you shall most likely not receive.* At the middle and high school level, guidance counselors are more uniformly available. However, the number of students they service may range from a manageable number, such that supportive services can be provided to students with greater needs, to one so large that no more than minimal clerical and scheduling duties can be performed. If the former is true at your child's school, her guidance counselor may be able to help you communicate more efficiently with teachers (by being the point person for the majority of school–home communication), meet one-on-one with your child, provide a "safe haven" if your child needs to temporarily exit a classroom, and help develop plans for accommodation.

SCHOOL PSYCHOLOGISTS

In most cases, a school psychologist will be shared by more than one school within a district. The primary role of the school psychologist is to conduct MFEs and to coordinate the development of IEPs. In some cases the school psychologist will be available to provide some group and individual therapy during school.

SCHOOL SOCIAL WORKER

A small number of schools have social workers on staff. Depending on the school, the role(s) played by a social worker will vary. He or she might provide some group and individual therapy, help to coordinate IEPs, work with families of students to foster better home–school communication, run whole-class programs, or consult with classroom teachers. Social workers may also serve as case managers for children who need a high level of services at school. Therapeutic schools and schools geared specifically to children with a high level of behavioral and emotional problems are most likely to have school social workers.

PRINCIPALS

Each school will have a principal and probably one or more assistant principals, depending on the size of the school. The primary function of a principal is administration. In smaller schools the principal might be integrally involved in the special education evaluation process and/or the development of the special education plan. Principals typically have the final say regarding the classroom in which each child is placed. Therefore, you might work with the principal to determine which of the third-grade teachers would make the best match for your very sensitive and anxious child or the best fifth-grade teacher for your spirited and sometimes explosive child.

SPECIAL EDUCATION COORDINATOR

This person typically serves more than one school in a district. Her function is to coordinate the team that determines which children need special education services and what services each child needs and to make sure that all children who need services are evaluated and receive the necessary services. This person is the administrator who oversees the special education teachers.

OCCUPATIONAL THERAPIST

Some schools will have their own occupational therapist (OT), some will share an OT among several schools, and some will hire an outside consultant to provide OT services to those children who need them. As part of your child's MFE, your child's fine motor skills may be assessed by an OT. This part of the evaluation will be conducted if problems have been noted by your child's classroom teacher. OTs help children develop their fine motor skills (e.g., those functions involved in writing and typing). OT services may be particularly helpful for children with graphomotor problems (e.g., difficulty writing) and should be specified in your child's IEP.

PHYSICAL THERAPIST

Whereas OTs focus on fine motor skills, physical therapists (PTs) work with children to develop gross motor skills and coordination. Again, this evaluation will be done if problems have been noted. Goals and objectives related to gross motor skills may be added to your child's IEP.

SPEECH/LANGUAGE PATHOLOGIST

Speech and language services will be added if your child has problems with verbal communication. These problems can range from articulation problems to difficulty forming and orally communicating ideas clearly. Your child's speech and language skills may be evaluated as part of her MFE.

OTHER SCHOOL PERSONNEL

When developing your child's IEP, we encourage you to think of every staff member in your child's building as a possible resource. Every school has its own special set of employees. People who work at schools tend to like kids. If you need some accommodations, start thinking creatively about who is available to assist. For example, the attendance coordinator, the in-school discipline specialist, or a member of the custodial or secretarial staff might be very helpful in meeting a unique need. Some ways in which we have encouraged families to use adjunctive school personnel include having an elementary school boy who had repeated conflicts during recess work as the custodian's assistant several days each week and having a middle school girl who was overwhelmed by lunch and recess assist in the main office during this time period. In both cases, the student gained esteem from providing meaningful assistance, while having a positive time with caring adults.

Getting Special Education Services

REQUEST A MEETING

A good place to start is with your child's teacher. Begin by sharing your concerns. Your child's teacher may have other observations. It is not uncommon for children with mood disorders to behave very differently at school than they do at home. Remember Marla, the ten-year-old with bipolar disorder Type II? She had periods of being a little bit giggly at school, but she was always careful to hide her irritability at school and with friends. Her teachers did not realize how difficult things were at home until they met with Marla's parents. On one hand, it was nice for Marla's parents to hear her teachers describe her in such glowing terms. On the other hand, hearing about how wonderful Marla was at school made them further question whether she needed treatment. Ultimately, Marla's parents opted for treatment because it became increasingly difficult for Marla to contain her moods at school and because she was having more and more difficulty at home.

When determining whom to approach first about an initial meeting, try to find someone who will make a comfortable contact for you. This should be someone who is accessible, who seems to have a good feel for your child's needs, and who makes you feel comfortable. This might be your child's teacher, the principal, the guidance counselor, or some other staff member. At the middle school and high school level, guidance counselors, team leaders, or homeroom teachers are sometimes the appropriate place to start.

BE PATIENT

If, based on your own research, as well as on consultation with your mental health team, you think your child needs services at school, request in writing that your child be evaluated. Be realistic and expect delays. Most school districts have waiting lists and testing takes considerable time and effort. However, the law specifies that a meeting to develop an IEP must be conducted within thirty days of determining special educational needs. Make sure you know who will lead the process and who will be involved. Ask for contact information so that you can stay informed. (See the Resources section for more detailed guides to walk you through this process.)

KEEP CAREFUL RECORDS (TAKE TWO)

This is a mantra to which we return again and again: Keep careful records. Keep copies of report cards, evaluation reports, and other documentation provided to you by the school. Whenever your child is evaluated (by the school or by private professionals), you should be given a written report. If one is not offered, ask! Remember the binder we suggested you keep in Chapter 4? Make sure it includes a section for school records. If your child needs extensive school services, you may need a separate binder just for school records.

WHAT IF THINGS GO WRONG?

Remember that evaluation findings are not final and that you do not have to accept the recommendations made by the educational team. You may appeal the conclusions. (This right is specified by the due process clause in IDEA, described in Table 5.) That said, remember to seek coalitions, not conflict, with your child's educational team.

Think Outside the Box: Educational Plans for Children with Mood Disorders

BE CREATIVE!

This may be the most important concept for helping your child adapt and in developing accommodations for your child. Here are some examples of special school accommodations arranged for children and adolescents with mood disorders. Their plans range from simple adjustments based on an agreement between teachers and parents to formal educational plans. You will find examples beginning at the preschool level and going up through high school. Although examples are provided for different grade levels, many of the ideas suggested transfer well across grade levels. (Drew, our first grader, experiences much relief from having a safe haven to which he can escape if he is feeling too stressed. This is a strategy we also employ with elementary, middle, and high school students.)

Carl, Preschool. Carl's mother, Susan, knew something was different about Carl from the day he was born. He never slept, walked at eight months, and has been constantly on the go ever since. His activity level is extremely difficult to manage at home and in his preschool class. He can be very aggressive and regularly has long and extreme tantrums. At times Carl's judgment is extremely poor. He once climbed the fence while his day care teacher wasn't looking. When she caught up with him, Carl was about to run into the street to "race a car because I'm faster than Superman." After several incidents of Carl hurting other children and also putting himself in danger, Carl's day care director suggested that he might need some educational services that they could not provide. The day care director helped Susan get in touch with the early childhood director for her home school district. An MFE was conducted, which involved an observation in Carl's current school setting, an interview with Susan, and some testing. Concurrently, Susan returned to Carl's pediatrician, who had been prescribing stimulant medication for Carl. When Susan described the problems Carl had been having, the pediatrician suggested a referral to a child and adolescent psychiatrist. A preschool IEP was developed for Carl. He began attending a specialized preschool class in the mornings, then he was transported (by bus, at the expense of his local school district) back to his regular day care center for lunch and rest time. Staff there agreed to continue working with Carl as long as they would have the support of his special education team. Carl saw his new psychiatrist, who started him on a mood stabilizer. With the benefits of his new medication and the support of his special class (which had a significantly smaller child–teacher ratio and activities tailored to meet his needs), Carl began to do better. His special education teacher helped Carl learn some skills to manage his anger, such as going to a special place in the class to calm himself down and asking a teacher to help him calm down. These same strategies were implemented at his day care center with considerable success.

Drew, First Grade. Drew is seven years old and in first grade. He has frequent episodes of tearfulness and gets frustrated and angry easily. At the beginning of the school year, Drew's parents, John and Amanda, requested a meeting with his teacher. John and Amanda explained that they had scheduled an appointment with a psychologist, but that they thought Drew might need some help at school right away. Drew's teacher invited the school guidance counselor to join the meeting, and they devised a plan for Drew. The guidance counselor offered her office as a place for Drew to go when he needed somewhere quiet to calm down. The principal's office was identified as a second possibility in case the guidance counselor was not available. They also set up an incentive system for Drew. Anytime the teacher noticed Drew handling his frustration appropriately (e.g., leaving the situation calmly, using words to express his feelings), she would put a star on a piece of paper. At the end of each day she would send that piece of paper home with a note to his parents about what he had done well. Drew's parents would reward him according to the number of stars on his daily paper. The teacher also planned to send an e-mail home describing any problems Drew had. Amanda would also send e-mails to Drew's teacher to keep her updated on his treatment progress and behavior at home and to provide a prompt for feedback on his behavior at school. After one month with this plan in place, Drew's parents met with his teacher again. Drew was having fewer episodes of tearfulness but was continuing to be easily frustrated by his peers. They agreed to have the school psychologist conduct a functional behavioral assessment (FBA) to see if she could identify any pattern to Drew's outbursts. The school psychologist noted that Drew tended to get upset when he and a peer were trying to negotiate the rules of a game or activity. Based on the school psychologist's observations, Drew's guidance counselor began spending some time in the classroom, especially during unstructured times, and tried to coach Drew through the process of initiating an activity. Social skills also became a focus of Drew's work with his new therapist.

Tisha, Third Grade. Tisha was diagnosed with dysthymic disorder at age seven and has recently been diagnosed with bipolar disorder-NOS and ADHD. She is frequently irritable, argues excessively with peers, and generally has a bad reputation with her classmates. She tends to invade peers' space and has no close friends at school. Although she has been tested and has an above-average IQ, Tisha is not doing well academically. She has particular difficulty with writing assignments and often fails to turn them in. Homework time is a daily struggle. When she showed no improvement after a month of school, Tisha's parents requested a meeting with her classroom teacher. The principal joined them at the meeting, because she had worked with Tisha several times following playground conflicts. They agreed that an MFE was needed and that Tisha was in need of special education services. The MFE revealed a written-language learning disability and documented significant emotional and behavioral problems. Tisha began to receive services from the SED resource room, the learning specialist, and the occupational therapist. She spent every morning with her regular class, then spent the afternoon in the resource room. This meant Tisha could have lunch and recess with the resource room teacher and thus receive significantly more support during that time. The occupational therapist began working with Tisha to address her significant difficulties with handwriting (graphomotor problems) by simultaneously working on her handwriting skills and her keyboarding skills.

Heather, Fifth Grade. Heather is an eleven-year-old who recently started taking lithium due to increasingly severe episodes of elevated mood, irritability, and grandiosity. Her symptoms were apparent primarily at home; her teachers had noticed only occasional periods of giddy behavior. Lithium has helped Heather be less irritable, think at a manageable pace, and make more realistic decisions. Overall, she is doing much better at home. Heather has always done well academically and has never had significant behavioral problems at school. Since starting lithium, however, Heather has to go to the bathroom frequently and is always thirsty. Heather was embarrassed to ask for the bathroom pass as often as she needed it, so her mother talked with her classroom teacher and arranged for Heather to be allowed to quietly leave the classroom and go to the bathroom between class periods. Since starting lithium, Heather has also been experiencing sedation that peaks just after lunch. This is typically when Heather's teacher gives the class time to work quietly on assignments or read silently. After Heather fell asleep at her desk twice, her teacher called home to request a meeting with Heather's parents. The teacher learned that sleepiness was a side effect of the medication that was likely to go away in time, and they arranged, on a temporary basis, for Heather to go to the nurse if she felt particularly sleepy. After two weeks, the sedation began to subside, and Heather was again able to use this quiet work time effectively.

Jacob, Seventh Grade. Jacob is twelve and hates school. Although Jacob grasps concepts easily, he is very disorganized and has considerable difficulty completing homework. When he does do his homework, he often forgets to turn it in. Jacob has grown increasingly irritable since the beginning of the school year, and his mother, Christina, has begun to wonder if his Prozac is still working and if his Adderall is helping enough. She was surprised when his report card showed a D average, because Jacob had told her he was doing "OK" and she hadn't heard from his teachers. Christina and her husband, Frank, requested a meeting with Jacob's teachers. Because the middle school had a team structure, they met with several members of the seventh-grade team, including the science teacher, who was the team leader. With the help of Jacob's guidance counselor, who was in charge of the school's Section 504 plans (see Table 4), they developed a 504 Plan that included weekly e-mail communication between Jacob's parents and Jacob's teachers. Frank and Christina would send an e-mail inquiring about missing work each Wednesday to Jacob's science teacher, who would check with Jacob's other teachers and respond by Thursday afternoon with a list of any missing assignments, so that Jacob could complete them over the weekend. The plan also specified that Jacob use an assignment notebook that would be checked and signed by his homeroom teacher each afternoon, then by his parents each evening. The 504 Plan would be put into place immediately. Additionally, a request was made to conduct an MFE. Meanwhile, Christina scheduled an appointment with Jacob's psychiatrist, who increased Jacob's dose of Prozac. He also suggested switching Jacob to a longer-acting formulation of Adderall (Adderall XR) to more effectively address Jacob's symptoms of ADHD (e.g., difficulty staying focused on homework, disorganization, forgetfulness, distractibility) throughout the school day.

Sherry, Ninth Grade. Sherry had become increasingly sad and had begun having panic attacks. After her boyfriend broke up with her, Sherry became despondent and took an overdose of an over-the-counter medication she found at home. Following this suicide attempt, Sherry was hospitalized for five days, then discharged on an antidepressant. Her parents were very concerned, they had not realized how serious Sherry's depression was until she attempted suicide. With the help of the hospital staff who started treatment, they arranged for Sherry to begin working as an outpatient with a therapist and to begin seeing a child and adolescent psychiatrist. Although Sherry was started on medication during her hospitalization, her recovery had only just begun. Prior to Sherry's returning to school, Sherry and her parents met with her guidance counselor. They arranged for Sherry to attend half days for the first two weeks, then to return to full days when she felt up to it. They would meet again prior to Sherry's returning to full days at school. The guidance counselor offered his office as a safe haven for Sherry whenever she felt she needed it. He also agreed to seek Sherry out each day to check in with her. Sherry did not want all of her teachers to know what had happened because she was afraid they would begin to treat her differently (Sherry had always been a good student and valued the respect of her teachers). Sherry did agree to tell her favorite teacher so that she could also look out for Sherry.

Luke, Eleventh Grade. Luke has never liked school and has always found it a struggle. Luke tends to be surly and withdrawn from his family, except when he is outside. He thrives on physical exertion and being close to nature. Luke was diagnosed with learning disabilities in reading and writing during elementary school. Ever since then, Luke has had resource-room support and access to a tutor. His older brother was an honor student and is currently a sophomore in college. Luke's parents, after fighting with Luke through elementary school, middle school, and the first half of high school, are tired of getting notices about Luke's not completing assignments and failing classes. Ready to give up, they requested a meeting with his guidance counselor. The guidance counselor suggested that Luke switch from a college-bound track to a vocational track. This would mean attending classes each morning but then going to a work site in the afternoons. Luke could graduate with his class and learn a viable trade. The guidance counselor thought they could arrange for an outdoor job site, possibly in carpentry. Although this was not what Luke's parents had envisioned for their younger son, a school program that Luke would be interested in and succeed in seemed preferable to their current daily battles. Luke agreed to the strict attendance and participation policies of the program and successfully graduated with his class.

Not all children with mood disorders need specialized services provided by the school, but many need help adjusting to school due to the impact of their mood symptoms. Schools are generally designed to meet

| TABLE 6 | Accommodations for Common Mood Disorder Related Problems |

Child's problem	Accommodation
Difficulty concentrating	Provide a quiet place to work, allow for headphones with quiet music.
Social withdrawal/ excessive peer conflict	Provide extra support from a teacher during recess and lunch, arrange "special time" with another staff person (e.g., janitor, office staff).
Difficulty staying focused during unstructured times	Increase structure, develop a buddy system if feasible.
Daily mood changes	Present most challenging activities during periods of most positive mood, increase teacher awareness of mood changes.
Frequent urination due to medication	Give permission for child to use the bathroom more frequently.
Fluctuations in energy level	Plan energizing activities for periods of fatigue, plan a daily rest period, design daily activity schedules to match child's typical activity level changes.

the needs of average children and adolescents with no special emotional, behavioral, or educational needs. Children with mood disorders do not fit this description particularly well and often have a range of special needs. To be the best possible advocate for your child at school, you need to understand your child's needs, learn about the available resources, request the appropriate services, and be ready to roll up your sleeves and tackle what may be a significant challenge.

At the beginning of this chapter we described some of the ways in which mood disorder symptoms may affect your child's functioning at school. As your child's advocate, part of your role is to help develop and request an accommodation plan. Some examples of requests you might make are included in Table 6. For further information, please refer to the reading materials and Web sites provided in our Resources section.

11 Crisis Management

As parents and heads of a household, you're probably well prepared for certain emergencies. Unfortunately, having a child with a mood disorder in the family can expand the list of crises that might occur. Not all children with mood disorders will have the types of crises described in this chapter, but we strongly encourage you to prepare for them anyway, both to minimize the damage wrought and to prevent you from panicking should an emergency arise.

There are two general categories of crisis management you should master: (1) ensuring safety in the face of out-of-control behavior such as violence and (2) managing specific challenging symptoms of mania and depression.

Ensuring Safety

For some children with mood disorders, the safety tips we describe here will never be required. For other children, these tips will need to be in place while they are at their worst but not after their episodes abate. We ask you to consider whether your child's behavior poses safety concerns. If so, we will help you develop a safety plan and a backup safety plan.

Think Ahead

If your child is prone to rages, don't wait until anger gets out of control to deal with safety issues. Stay ahead of the symptoms if at all possible. Review the following list to address the potential dangers that might be present in your home/daily life.

- *Knives.* How can you secure kitchen knives? Possibilities include locking knives in a car trunk, placing them in a lockable pantry, or installing a padlock on a kitchen drawer.
- *Guns.* Studies have proven that it is not sufficient to lock up guns in one portion of the home and to lock up the ammunition in another portion of the home. *Get them out of the house.* (This is *not* an antigun statement; this is a prosafety statement.)
- *Transportation.* How will you transport your child if he can't sit safely in a car (e.g., he is trying to jump out of the moving car)? Can another adult ride with you? Do you need to call the police or an ambulance service? If traffic safety is an issue, how can it be managed?
- *Therapeutic holds.* To keep yourself and your child safe, know how to hold your child if she is a danger to herself or others. Also know when it is not safe (or will make the situation worse) to attempt physically restraining your child or teenager.
- *Door locks.* Installing locks on bedroom doors for siblings can be very important, because siblings are often are targets of hostility. Siblings need a safe place within the home to which they can retreat. You will want to ensure that the sibling knows how to unlock the door and that you always have a way to unlock the door.

Emergency Treatment and Hospitalization

When Andy, Carmen's seven-year-old son, grabbed a knife during a particularly violent rage and threatened his younger sister, Carmen was well prepared. She quickly made a phone call to her brother-in-law, Jim, who lived two blocks away and had agreed to be her backup if she ever needed help. Jim's arrival surprised Andy enough that he dropped the knife and returned to lying on the kitchen floor, kicking and screaming. Carmen called Andy's psychiatrist and told her what was happening. The doctor advised Carmen to take Andy to the emergency room. Carmen had contacted her insurance company previously and knew to which emergency room she should take Andy. Further, she knew that her insurance would cover the only local child and adolescent psychiatric unit (in Carmen's case, as is the case in many communities, there is only one child and adolescent psychiatric hospital in the area). Carmen called her neighbor and arranged for her to take care of Andy's sister. Then, with Jim sitting in the back seat with Andy, she drove to the hospital with her binder of information about Andy's treatment on the seat next to her.

Carmen did everything right. She was in a situation with Andy that was extremely frightening, but because she had prepared in advance, she could go on "automatic pilot" and did not need to problem-solve on the spot. If you've organized the binder we've been recommending throughout this book, you already have much of the information you should have accessible in case of a crisis in one place. Some of this information should also be shared with school personnel, in case crises occur at school.

Your crisis information file should include:

1. Emergency phone numbers:
   - Family or friends to help manage your child or take care of siblings; have daytime and evening contact numbers
   - Your prescribing physician and therapist; have both business and after-hours numbers
2. Medication information
   - Complete listing of medication names, dosages, and times administered
   - Fact sheets that describe side effects and how to handle them
3. Hospitalization information
   - Address of hospital (and directions to get there)
   - Insurance coverage, including inpatient preauthorization requirements

Contacting the Police

Many communities rely on the police to handle mental health emergencies. The skill with which emergencies are handled varies widely. You should know when and how to contact your local police. As a general rule of thumb, if you think you might need to call the police due to the severity of your child's symptoms, you should also proactively develop a mental health team. They can give you guidelines regarding what other local resources (e.g., a twenty-four-hour crisis center) may be more appropriate or to which you can have the police escort you and your child.

You may find the idea of calling the police very frightening, especially if you don't know what to expect if you do call. Many police departments have a juvenile officer whose main function is to work with youth and their families. Often these officers are highly skilled, connect well with children, and are very supportive of parents. Sometimes such personnel are not available, however. To find out what you might encounter and so that you can explain in advance that your child has a volatile and unpredictable illness, consider making an advance visit or phone call to the juvenile officer at your local police station. You'll feel a lot better if you know up front how a crisis, such as your child's becoming dangerous and impossible for you to manage, might be handled.

We can't stress enough, however, the importance of consulting your mental health team for advice on preparing for and handling emergencies such as Carmen's. Your local treatment team can tell you what resources are available within your community that are appropriate for your child's unique needs. For example, parents can and do press charges against their children in extreme cases of repeated, unrelenting violence, but clearly the court system is not a good choice in all situations. In communities that do not have a mental health court or a sophisticated juvenile justice program, pressing charges could backfire, causing your child to end up in a placement that is not therapeutic and is potentially damaging.

Ten-year-old Steven has been a handful for his mother, Kathy, almost since he was born. Steven's father has bipolar disorder but will not remain in treatment. When Kathy was pregnant, he became manic and physically assaultive toward Kathy. As a result, Kathy divorced Steven's father before Steven was born. His father has not attempted to be a regular part of Steven's life, about which Kathy feels relieved. However, Steven was also diagnosed with bipolar disorder by the time he turned seven. Although Steven has very limited contact with his father, Kathy is struck by the uncanny resemblances Steven has to him. One of the least endearing is Steven's similar dislike for taking his medication on a regular basis. Although Kathy has tried to talk to Steven about the importance of taking his medications, Steven is clever about hiding his pills and not swallowing them. Steven has repeatedly been aggressive toward Kathy and destructive to property during episodes of rage. During a particularly violent rage, Steven kicked Kathy in the stomach, and she chose to call the police. She had repeatedly warned her son that she would call the police if he hurt her, as she had been encouraged to do by Steven's case manager, and this time she decided she had to follow through. Seeing his mother fulfill her threat shocked Steven enough that he calmed down slightly, and when two police officers arrived within minutes of the call, his rage ceased.

Also with the encouragement of Steven's mental health team, Kathy pressed assault charges against her son. Steven appeared in juvenile court and was placed on probation. His probation officer met with him weekly at school and came to the house periodically. Steven was also enrolled in an anger management program through the juvenile court.

Meanwhile, Kathy was instructed to call the probation officer if Steven was ever aggressive toward her.

Again, this recourse is not appropriate in all cases or in all places. Kathy turned to the police not at the first hint of trouble but only after a long and painful (figuratively and literally) struggle with Steven and his difficulties. She decided on this course of action only because her case manager was intimately familiar with local resources and could help Kathy connect to programs that work well within her community. Kathy and Steven live in a community in which the juvenile justice system is well developed, and alternative sentencing (probation with a probation officer savvy about children with mental health issues and enrollment in an anger management course) is available.

As it turned out, being held accountable for his behavior encouraged Steven to find other, more appropriate outlets for his anger. Through his anger management course, he learned to recognize the triggers that often led to his becoming very angry. He also began to understand that he tended to take his anger out on his mother rather than seeking her assistance to calm down. Prior to being placed on probation, Steven had attended therapy, but it had never been very helpful because he was unwilling to take responsibility for his actions. Steven began to acknowledge his illness and to accept that, despite his illness, inappropriate and especially dangerous behavior was not going to be tolerated. As a result he started to take his medication more willingly. This approach worked for Kathy and Steven because she had worked with her mental health team in advance on exploring all the possible alternatives and had been diligent in matching available resources with Steven's needs.

Managing Challenging Symptoms

Throughout this book we provide suggestions for dealing with symptoms of depression and mania. Because, however, manic episodes have some unique features that can drive a family to crisis, here we offer several specific tips for managing mania.

Managing Manic Episodes

STAY AHEAD OF THE GAME

One challenge for parents of children with bipolar disorder is to stay one step ahead of the disorder. If you can recognize the early stages of mania, you can deploy resources to try to stop the mania in its tracks. Don't allow yourself to get carried away with a "high" mood. If your child experiences a euphoric mood when manic, the early stages of mania can seem pleasant or fun, especially if your child has recently been sad or irritable. Recognize the need for treatment and activate your treatment team.

AVOID MAKING MATTERS WORSE

If you can, avoid highly stimulating situations, such as staying until the end of a large family party that would involve keeping your child up well past her bedtime. Temporarily take away privileges that could get your child into trouble or create safety hazards. If, for example, your child is allowed to be home alone after school, arrange for someone to be home with him. If your teenager likes to go shopping at the mall and has access to a debit card, take it away from her.

Julia, now twelve, had been doing well on a combination of a mood stabilizer, a low dose of an antidepressant, and a stimulant for co-occurring ADHD for about a year when her mother, Elaine, started to notice a change. Julia was giggling a lot, had some excess energy, and was really interested in starting several new activities. Julia wasn't doing poorly, but Elaine saw the writing on the wall and called Julia's psychiatrist, who asked that Elaine schedule an appointment for Julia and also take her for a blood draw prior to her appointment to check Julia's Depakote level. Elaine also found an excuse to cancel a late-night event they were supposed to attend over the upcoming weekend.

DON'T ARGUE

If the early stages of mania have progressed, carefully manage the later stages. Don't argue with your child's assertion that she is the smartest person in her whole school. You won't win, and you're likely to be met by an ugly response.

BACK TO BUSINESS

Once the episode has passed, go back to "business as usual," but go slowly. Mania is an illness and needs recovery time like any other illness. Adding too much too soon may precipitate further problems.

As Mark, thirteen, became more and more manic, he became more and more difficult to live with. He was argumentative and impulsive, and everything he said seemed outrageously exaggerated. It was tempting for his mother, Janice, to correct his misstatements, but she kept remembering his therapist's advice: "Don't argue with him when he is irrational. You won't win." Instead, she tried to keep things as calm as possible at home and keep faith that the increases in his medications would start to help soon. Janice was eager to get life back to normal and to get Mark back into his regular routine. She knew that she would need his treatment team's support and guidance to determine the pace at which they could get back to business as usual.

LET BYGONES BE BYGONES

After the manic episode, don't unnecessarily humiliate your child by reminding him or her about manic behavior. However, if your child is resisting treatment and refusing to acknowledge that there is a problem, reminders about manic behavior may be necessary.

Antoine, sixteen, was recently released from the hospital after being stabilized for a severe episode of mania that was accompanied by psychosis. Prior to hospitalization, Antoine believed he had special powers, offered to "make his services available" to his boss at the diner where he works as a waiter, and heard voices telling him that he should run for mayor of his town. Now that Antoine has been stable for several months, he is annoyed by the side effects of his medication and has decided that he won't take it anymore, because he is doing well and he doesn't have any problems. Antoine does not recall all of his unusual beliefs and out-of-control behaviors that occurred prior to and during his hospitalization. His father, Kenneth, had been told by the unit social worker not to refer back to Antoine's symptoms during hospitalization. However, Kenneth is worried sick that Antoine's refusal to take medication will result in the recurrence of his symptoms. With the assistance of Antoine's outpatient case manager, Kenneth gently reminded Antoine of the problems that led to hospitalization. Antoine had not remembered all the details of his behavior until this conversation. Fear of embarrassing himself at work again helped convince him to continue with his medications as prescribed.

Managing Suicide Threats and Attempts

According to the Centers for Disease Control and Prevention in Atlanta, each year approximately 2 million teenagers in America attempt suicide, and nearly 700,000 receive medical attention after these attempts. Suicidal ideation is even more common—as many as one in four high school girls and one in six high school boys have had serious thoughts about suicide in the previous twelve-month period.

We know that mood disorders (both depression and bipolar disorder) place children and teenagers at heightened risk for suicidal behavior, including suicide attempts. We also know that effective treatment of the mood disorder (and any accompanying conditions) is the best antidote for suicidal behavior. So being kept informed about suicidal thoughts is nine-tenths of the battle. You need to know the risk factors for and warning signs of suicidal behavior. We also need to debunk the common misconception that asking someone whether he is experiencing suicidal thoughts might give him ideas about making a suicide attempt. The opposite is actually true. By asking directly when you're concerned, you convey your care for your child and your awareness that suicidal thoughts might be on his or her mind and that you plan to stay on top of what's going on and thus can help maintain safety. The greatest danger is ignoring warning signs (see sidebar). If you notice any of these warning signs, your child should be working with mental health professionals who should be made aware of these worrisome behaviors.

First and foremost, take suicidal talk and gestures seriously. Suicidal gestures are self-destructive or self-harming behaviors that are not life threatening but may indicate that a child is thinking about suicide. Examples of suicidal gestures include scratching one's wrist

---

TIPS FOR PARENTS: SUICIDE RISKS AND WARNING SIGNS

Suicidal thoughts and behaviors are most likely to occur:

1. During or right after inpatient treatment
2. During a crisis
3. Following the suicide of a close friend or relative
4. Around positive or negative life events

Warning signs include:

1. Talking about death or suicide
2. Saying good-byes
3. Making wills
4. Giving away belongings

Other risk factors include:

1. Depressed or hopeless feelings
2. Drug and alcohol use
3. Impulsivity
4. Angry feelings
5. Physical or sexual abuse
6. Being a runaway
7. Past attempt(s)
8. A history of self-destructive behavior
9. Being perfectionistic
10. Having access to guns

and taking a few pills (not enough to be life threatening but more than the recommended dose).

The myth that suicidal talk is just a way to get attention is a particularly dangerous one. There are two possibilities. Either the suicidal talk is an indication of intention to act, or it is a cry for help. Either way, attention *is* needed. Pay attention to reckless behavior. A child who has displayed some other risk factors and also rides his bike in a dangerous manner may be crying out for help.

If you suspect suicidal thoughts, start by increasing supervision. Remove available methods such as medications and guns. Know how and when to access the emergency room and hospitalization. Discuss these concerns with your child's treatment team. Find out from them when and how they recommend you take action (e.g., taking your child to an emergency department or crisis management center).

We cannot prepare you for every possible emergency, but we can encourage you to think carefully about your child, the course of your child's illness so far, the potential dangers in your home, your resources, and your community's resources. Preplanning for a crisis will allow you to keep a cool head if a stressful situation occurs. It may even help to de-escalate a situation if you can (relatively) calmly outline to your child the subsequent steps you will need to take if the crisis behavior does not abate.

Part IV

Helping Your Family Live with a Mood Disorder

We don't have to tell you that a child's mood disorder can affect family life in numerous ways, from wreaking havoc with normal family cycles and patterns to causing resentment in siblings to wearing out the adults in charge. Too often these problems get put on a back burner while you deal with the more urgent tasks of managing the child's depressive and manic episodes and keeping the child functioning. In the following chapters we tell you how to rescue the entire family from the clutches of one child's mood disorder.

When you're immersed in day-to-day management of mood symptoms, the negative family cycles that commonly occur in families struggling with a mood disorder often escape notice. But these cycles can be avoided with a slight shift in attention and a few positive steps taken within your family, as explained in Chapter 12. Siblings often bear the brunt of a child's mood symptoms. Not infrequently they are the targets of aggression and displays of temperament. They end up feeling neglected and underappreciated. In Chapter 13 we alert you to common emotional reactions that you'll want to be on the lookout for in your other children and offer tips for supporting these innocent bystanders to mood disorders. Finally, in the "last but definitely not least" category, we focus on *you* in Chapter 14. Your child's mood disorder can be exhausting and depleting, and in this chapter we ask you to follow some simple suggestions for taking care of yourself while you're taking care of everyone else.

12 How Mood Disorders Affect Family Life

Until now, we have explored how your child's mood disorder affects *her* life—at home, at school, and with others her age. However, children live within families. This means that your child's mood disorder will have a significant impact on your family as a whole, as well as on siblings and on you and your spouse or partner. In this chapter we describe how your child's mood disorder can set negative cycles into motion and how you can interrupt those cycles with positive interactions. Specifically, we focus on how to create a balance for you, your child, and your family and how to fight stigma and isolation.

First, an important caveat. The fact that you're reading this book makes it clear that you care greatly about your child and your family and that you want the best for everyone, individually and collectively. Unfortunately, there is no such thing as the perfect family or the perfect home life, mood disorder or no mood disorder. You'll do the best you can, some things will fall through the cracks, you'll have good aspects of family life and some not so good ones, there will be good days and bad days. That's OK. In trying to manage and nurture an entire family, it's more important than ever that you set aside crippling self-blame.

Negative Family Cycles

All families of children with mood disorders are unique, and all will experience the challenges of raising a moody child in their own particular ways. However, some patterns and experiences are common to many families. We frequently hear about what we and others refer to as the "negative family cycle." This cycle includes a series of well-intentioned actions, negative reactions, and hurt feelings. This cycle was originally described by Diane Holder and Carol Anderson from the University of Pittsburgh in a discussion of how to help adults with mood disorders. We have applied the ideas to families of children with mood disorders. The cycle starts with the family trying to help by coaxing, reassuring, and protecting. The child or adolescent doesn't respond positively to this. The family reacts either by trying even harder or by withdrawing. Often each parent attempts a different solution, and parental attention turns to criticizing the other parent's ineffective solution. Meanwhile, although the child or teenager feels some relief from "getting off the hook," he also feels more alienated, and parents feel rejected. At this point, without intervention, the family can fall deeper into this negative cycle— with parents either withdrawing from the child or getting angry or doing both. Again, it is common for parents to take on different roles and then to fight with each other. From this point, parents often feel guilty and go back to coaxing, reassuring, and protecting. The child feels increasingly unworthy, hopeless, and infantilized. Over time parents burn out but still feel guilty and/or angry. The end result is that the child feels alienated and/or overprotected. This cycle, or parts of it, tends to repeat until a significant change is made to alter it.

Tom and Marsha started having trouble with their son Griffin when he was an infant. Difficult to get to sleep at night, Griffin had stopped taking naps when he was two and had always seemed temperamental and prickly. But things had really come to a head when Griffin was twelve and began to have more and more periods of irritability. Convinced that the stresses of school were the cause, Marsha spent hours with her son each afternoon, helping him and encouraging him to complete his homework. Being a twelve-year-old boy and being particularly irritable in the afternoons, Griffin found his mother's efforts annoying and was often rude and surly to her. Tom thought Marsha was babying Griffin too much and repeatedly told her to back off and let him experience the natural consequences of not completing his work. At the same time, Tom couldn't stand to hear Griffin be so rude to his mother, so he'd get angry and insist that his son act nicer; in turn, Griffin would get frustrated with his father, as well. Fed up with Griffin's lack of positive response and irritability, Tom withdrew. Marsha felt unsupported but pressed ahead with trying to help and protect Griffin. She became increasingly upset with Tom's lack of involvement, which led to arguments between Tom and Marsha. This continued with Marsha feeling like she was fighting for her family while Tom spent longer hours at work to avoid being at home.

Finally, Marsha confided in a good friend from her teaching days. Her friend listened to her descriptions of Griffin's moods and suggested that he might benefit from seeing a therapist. Marsha followed through. Griffin was diagnosed with cyclothymia and began taking a mood stabilizer. He also started working with a therapist, who focused both on helping Griffin to build his own coping strategies and on helping the family to learn to cope. Marsha and Tom learned that the patterns of responding they had tried were very typical but very damaging to themselves as a couple, not to mention that their disagreements led to ineffective parenting. They developed strategies together with which they were both comfortable. Tom and Marsha, with the help of the therapist, clarified for each other the positive intention of their actions, even though the actions themselves had backfired. They also learned to recognize each other's strengths. For example, there are some situations that Marsha is better equipped to manage (she's great at helping Griffin negotiate social dilemmas), whereas Tom can better handle other conflicts (Tom is skillful in helping Griffin figure out how to manage his own symptoms, as we saw in Chapter 9). Now fourteen, Griffin is functioning better at home and at school. Tom and Marsha are supporting each other and respecting each other's role with their son, and they are alert to the negative cycles that can impose themselves on their family at any time due to the stress of their son's mood disorder.

Griffin's family provides an example of how negative cycles caused by mood symptoms can sneak into a family and mess up relationships and life in general. Tom and Marsha have a fundamentally strong marriage. They are committed to their children and want to do what is best for them. Nevertheless, Griffin's mood disorder took over their family for a period of time. Identifying the mood disorder and initiating treatment broke the cycle. We hope that reading this book will help you identify and rectify the negative cycles that are affecting your family.

Keeping a Balance

Tom and Marsha recognized that they were in a negative family cycle and took steps to break it. Here are some additional ideas you can use to keep a healthy balance and avoid that negative cycle within your own family.

To Each His Own

Part of interrupting negative cycles is finding a balance for yourself, your family, and your child. You will be more apt to find balance if you recognize that each family member experiences a different reality. Recognizing and accepting those realities, or gently helping to revise them, is an important process. Your child and his or her siblings are likely to see things only from their own perspective.

Kevin is ten and his sister, Abby, is eight. Kevin complains that he is always picked on (he is frequently kept from watching TV as a result of being rude to family members). Abby complains that Kevin always gets his way and that she never gets to do what she wants to do.

In addition to the children in the house seeing things differently, you and your spouse may have your own perspectives. Acknowledging those differences may help you to form a more united front. It's particularly important to recognize that no perspective is wrong. You may see your child as needing treatment and support, whereas your spouse may see your child as needing consistency and firm discipline. You could interpret this as a major disagreement or, instead, acknowledge that you *both* are correct. Your child needs treatment, support, consistency, and discipline, but you choose to emphasize support and treatment whereas your spouse acknowledges the need for treatment but also emphasizes firm discipline.

Agree to Disagree

At times, you and your partner may simply not agree on an issue. In that case, you will need to "agree to disagree." When this happens, we suggest you use the problem-solving steps described in Chapter 8 to build in an evaluation period for Parent A's solution. If it doesn't work, then you agree to shift to Parent B's solution. If that doesn't work either, then the two of you will need to put your heads together to come up with a third solution.

Getting Seth, age nine, dressed in the morning is a daily challenge. He wakes up grumpy and is very difficult to get moving. Kathy, his mother, tends to handle him in the morning by gently teasing him and playfully getting him through the dressing process. Unfortunately, this sometimes takes up to thirty minutes of her morning. Tim, Seth's father, thinks Seth is old enough to get dressed independently and be ready for school on time. He finds this process incredibly frustrating to watch and sometimes steps in to help. His approach is to threaten Seth with losing privileges if he is not ready within a certain time limit. This approach sometimes gets Seth dressed more quickly but more often leads to tears and to Seth losing privileges. Kathy and Tim have had numerous arguments related to the morning routine. Finally they brought the situation up with their family therapist, Dr. Barr, who suggested that they agree to disagree. Kathy would take responsibility for getting Seth dressed, and Tim would go downstairs, have breakfast with their two older children, read the newspaper, and drink his coffee. If, after two weeks of this solution, Kathy was tired of her role, she could ask to switch with Tim. Dr. Barr's only additional comment was that Kathy and Tim needed to clearly let Seth know which plan was in place ahead of time, so that he could be prepared for the consequences. Seth's initial response to this problem when it was raised was that he "couldn't help" not getting up. In a family session Dr. Barr suggested that Seth could suggest a Plan C if he, his mom, and his dad weren't satisfied with Plan A or Plan B. As long as Seth's parents were willing to go along with whatever Plan C Seth concocted, they could try that next.

Remember, the Disorder Is Not the Child

It's easiest to avoid a negative cycle within the family when you keep your child's symptoms separate from your child in your mind. By definition, childhood-onset mood disorders occur prior to the full formation of personality or self-identity, so keeping these concepts clearly distinct can be challenging at times, if not impossible. Nevertheless, knowing your child's symptoms and recognizing their impact on you and on family life can only help. Periodically review your child's strengths and involve your child in that process (see the "Naming the Enemy" exercise in Chapter 2).

Don't Turn into an Analyst!

Trying to figure out *why* your child is depressed is a natural response to your child's misery. Being aware of environmental triggers that can set off symptoms is an important skill for you to have and for your child to develop. However, if you attempt to understand every nuance of your child's condition, it will only lead to frustration or guilt. Children, and teenagers in particular, tell us that they appreciate their parents conveying support and concern, but they hate their parents' trying to "become their therapist." Remember the container analogy we presented in Chapter 8? If you put your energy into letting your child know you care about his feelings, your child is more likely to share his feelings again at a later date than if you pry into his every experience and try to understand his feelings on a daily basis. It's also helpful to recognize that depression does not always have an environmental cause. In fact, many children have told us they feel guilty about being depressed because they recognize that they have a good life and don't know why they feel so bad.

Recognize Needs of All Family Members

Research has shown us that mood disorders tend to run in families. This means that parents of children with mood disorders frequently have mood disorders themselves. Often parents aren't themselves in treatment when they bring their children in to us for evaluations. For some parents, reviewing diagnostic criteria for their children makes them realize that the troubles they've been experiencing could also be due to a mood disorder of their own. Some other parents are reluctant to seek treatment on their own because they don't like the idea of going to see "just anybody." After we get to know these parents through our work with their child, they can benefit from a referral to a well-matched clinician. Finally, many families have heard horror stories about family members receiving ineffective treatment in the past, which discourages them from seeking treatment for themselves (even if they recognize the problems with which they are dealing). When these parents seek consultation for their child, the therapist has the opportunity to educate these parents about more contemporary treatments, which have improved dramatically in the past twenty-five years. Trying to parent a child with a mood disorder if you have an untreated mood disorder yourself is like having your hands tied behind your back and being blindfolded, then being put into the center of the room and told to pin the tail on the donkey. It's a pretty impossible task to get done right.

Once you've managed to identify and avoid the negative family cycle trap and you've developed healthy ways to maintain balance within your home, it's time to address issues that extend beyond the four walls of your home.

Dealing with Stigma

Unfortunately, mental illness continues to carry considerable stigma in our society. You may have had the experience of avoiding family or community gatherings due to concern about how your son's or daughter's behavior might be perceived. You may have also hesitated to share information about your child's or teen's illness with friends or family members for similar reasons. So whom should you tell? The school? Your friends? Your family members?

The answer varies. Who, what, and when to tell is a very personal decision. Older children and teenagers, whether they have a mood disorder themselves or whether they are a sibling of the child with a mood disorder, should also be involved in the decision. If safety is a concern or if your child or teen is likely to need extra support at school, sharing information with the school may be critical to your child's success. Your decision about whom to tell at the school might be based on who seems to know your child best or on who makes you feel comfortable. Depending on your situation, you might choose to tell your child's classroom teacher, your teen's guidance counselor, or the school principal. Keep in mind that schools function like small towns, and even if you tell only one person at school, other school staff will no doubt also become aware of this information. If you have special concerns about confidentiality (e.g., for the sake of a sibling), you're entitled to make these concerns known to the person in whom you initially confide.

Deciding whether to tell friends and family may require a lot of thought on your part. Are family members likely to be supportive? Have you noticed other family members struggling with similar problems (e.g., does your nephew's behavior remind you of your daughter's behavior before she started treatment)? Unlike family, you do get to choose your friends, and you need your friends as a source of support and comfort. It may not be appropriate to tell all of your friends, but having some friends who understand and are supportive may be really helpful in the long run.

The most damaging aspect of stigma is the isolation it causes. So, in addition to seeking support from friends and family, try to connect to community resources for support. Community agencies such as the local chapter of the National Alliance for the Mentally Ill (NAMI) and local Mental Health Associations (MHA) are geared toward providing support for individuals with mental illnesses and their family members, and they provide assistance with finding a variety of resources. Additionally, the

SHOULD I APPLY FOR SOCIAL SECURITY?

- The Social Security Administration (SSA) provides benefits in the form of *Supplemental Security Income* (SSI) for disabled children whose families have limited income and resources.
- To be eligible for SSI, your child must have a medically proven physical or mental condition that results in marked and severe functional limitations. This condition must last or be expected to last at least twelve months or be expected to result in death. The child can't be working at a job considered to be "substantial."
- Children who qualify for SSI also qualify for Medicaid, a health program for people with low income and limited assets.
- Continuing Disability Review (CDR) is required every three years for recipients under eighteen whose conditions are likely to improve and not later than twelve months after birth for babies whose disability is based on low birth weight.

amount of support on the World Wide Web is increasing dramatically. In particular, CABF provides free on-line support groups. (See the Resources section for information on how to contact community agencies and Internet support services).

We hope this chapter has helped to raise your awareness of some general issues that families of children with mood disorders face. We recognize the need to prioritize—you will need to take some time to address the most impairing symptoms of your child's mood disorder before you can turn to dealing with other issues. Once you've reached the point at which you feel that your child's symptoms are manageable or at least on the mend, it will be helpful for you to step back to determine how the mood disorder is affecting your overall family life, your ability to co-parent, yourself, your spouse, and your other children. Negative family cycles are a frequent experience of families raising moody children. But there are ways to get "unstuck." You can help your family by recognizing the cycles, acknowledging and allowing the different perspectives of family members, striving for balance, getting treatment for those who need it (including family therapy), separating the child from the disorder, and accessing support as a way of fighting stigma.

13 | How Can You Help Siblings?

Siblings of children with mood disorders experience a wide range of feelings—and often experience mixed feelings in response to their mentally ill sibling. The feelings range from fear, anger, and bitterness to embarrassment, loneliness, and isolation. Siblings sometimes feel resentful, burdened by trying to compensate for their ill sibling, and guilty for being healthy. Siblings also struggle with jealousy and feeling as though they are unimportant.

Sibling Conflicts

Debbie and Jason

Debbie is seven and often the target of Jason's aggression during manic episodes. Jason, who is ten, has experienced manic symptoms since he was three. During rages Jason has chased Debbie with a stick in hand, thrown chairs at her, and caused her numerous bruises. Their parents are supportive but have not always been able to protect Debbie from her brother's mood-related aggression. Sometimes Debbie gets so angry at Jason that she feels like hurting him. He has destroyed so many of her things. Just last week he ruined her social studies project by scribbling on the poster she had been working on for several days. At times like these Debbie does things to get even with Jason. Debbie's parents get frustrated with her because she instigates fights at times when Jason is calm. This usually results in Debbie getting in trouble, causing her to feel more bitter than ever.

Cynthia and Chloe

Cynthia is fourteen. Her younger sister, Chloe, is eleven and has bipolar disorder. Although Chloe is fairly stable now—she is on a good combination of medications and has an excellent therapist—she continues to be silly at the wrong moments, bosses peers around, and argues about everything. On the other hand, Cynthia is a good student and is well liked by everyone. Cynthia has watched her sister make a fool of herself over and over again. She is frustrated by and disgusted with Chloe, who never seems to know how to act and doesn't seem to learn from her mistakes. Cynthia is embarrassed by Chloe's behavior at school and in public and is worried that people will think there is something wrong with her because of her sister. Cynthia avoids having friends come to her house. As a result, she often feels lonely and isolated from her peers. To top it off, their parents spend a large amount of their afternoon and early evening time, as well as money, taking Chloe to her many appointments.

Dave and Nick

Dave is nine, and his brother, Nick, is fourteen. Nick is frequently irritable, spends a lot of time alone in his room, and has little energy. From Dave's perspective, Nick is rude and lazy, yet everyone seems to walk around on eggshells just to keep him happy. Nick doesn't do his chores, so Dave is asked to do extra. He resents the dark cloud that Nick frequently brings to the family. Dave feels bad for his mother, who often bears the brunt of Nick's wrath, so he tries not to be any trouble. And yet Dave sees that Nick is unhappy, that he doesn't have any friends, and that he has a hard time doing his schoolwork. Dave feels bad for Nick and a little bit guilty when he gets invited to a birthday party or brings home a good report card.

Joey and Krista

Joey, six, couldn't believe it when his sister, Krista, ten, came in carrying a toy from a Happy Meal. Why does she always get to go to McDonald's when he gets stuck eating meat loaf at Grandma's? Why doesn't he get to spend time with Mom and go out to dinner? Joey's resentment comes out in his teasing and taunting his sister, calling her a "baby" and making faces at her whenever his parents can't see him. Krista nearly always tattles on him, and Joey ends up being punished. Life seems so unfair to Joey.

It's Not All Negative

The feelings that siblings of children with mood disorders experience run the gamut. However, they are not always negative. When Jason is more stable, he can be very funny and can really get Debbie laughing. If Cynthia sees Chloe being teased on the playground, she immediately comes to her rescue. Before Nick got so depressed, he was a really good drummer. Every now and then he will sit back down at his drum set and jam. Dave thinks his brother is just the coolest when he does that. One time, after teasing Krista, Joey heard her in her room saying, "Why am I so stupid? Who could ever like me? Even my little brother thinks I'm a jerk!" Joey felt so bad, he racked his brain to think of what nice thing he could do for Krista to cheer her up.

What Can Parents Do?

The first step for parents is to remember that siblings have needs, too. The tough job is finding the emotional resources within yourself to deal with them. We address ways to do that shortly. Returning to the siblings, however, the first step is recognizing that siblings also need support. Simply conveying to your other children that you acknowledge that they, too, have feelings and reactions to their brother's or sister's difficulties goes a long way. Siblings benefit from getting a clear message that not only are mixed or negative emotions OK but that they are also normal and predictable. Helping siblings accept negative feelings they have toward their brother or sister may also help you recognize and accept similar feelings in yourself.

Second, parents will do well to realize that they can't meet every need of every family member. Whether you're in a single- or a dual-parent household, when the child with the mood disorder is demanding attention, you probably feel short-staffed in the adult department. It is, of course, precisely at these times that siblings need the most support. For that reason you can help siblings by nurturing the relationships they have with one or more adults outside the home who can provide support and be positive role models. These other adults could include a school guidance counselor, youth minister, grandmotherly neighbor, Big Brother or Big Sister, close family friend, or special relative.

More ideas for what you can do to help your other children follow.

Recognize and Manage Common Problems

After acknowledging their feelings and fostering relationships, you can take additional steps to help your other children. They may or may not need assistance in every category we've listed, but reading through this section will help increase your awareness of the types of difficulties your other children might be experiencing and what you can do to support them.

MENTAL HEALTH TREATMENT NEEDS

Full and half siblings share family history, so they are also at increased risk for mood disorders, as well as any co-occurring problems, such as anxiety, behavior, or learning disorders, that their mood-impaired brother or sister has. When one family member's symptoms are particularly severe, it's easy to miss less severe problems in other members. As a result, these difficulties can remain hidden for long periods of time. In addition, younger siblings may not begin to manifest symptoms until they reach a particular age. Your job as a parent is to respond to symptoms as best you can when you notice them. It can be particularly difficult to acknowledge and accept mood symptoms in a child who is "the healthy one." We address issues related to grief and acceptance further in Chapter 14.

Grace is ten, in the fifth grade, and is the younger sister of thirteen-year-old Robert, who was diagnosed with major depressive disorder (MDD) two years ago. Grace had always done well in school. When Grace brought home her second-quarter report card, her mother, Yvette, was stunned. Grace had all C's and D's as compared to her typical A's and B's. Yvette immediately sat down to talk with Grace. She learned that Grace had been feeling down, having trouble sleeping, and struggling to concentrate. Yvette called Robert's therapist, who helped schedule an evaluation for Grace with another clinician in the practice. Based on the evaluation, Grace started therapy. The clinician, in conjunction with Grace's parents, decided to monitor her closely. If her depressive symptoms did not subside with therapy, they would reevaluate the possibility of starting medication.

ACTING OUT

When children experience the strong mixed feelings that come with having a sibling with a mood disorder, they sometimes respond by acting out. Acting out may be a way of expressing anger, resentment, or jealousy or may be a sibling's way of "trying out" the behaviors that seem to attract parental attention to their sibling. Debbie is sick of Jason's bipolar disorder. Currently his mood is fairly stable, and he's doing well. When Debbie's mother asked her to set the table one evening, Debbie threw herself on the floor and started screaming. Her mother, surprised by her behavior, sent Debbie to her room. On her way there, Debbie slammed two doors and stomped up the stairs so hard that the floor shook. Later that evening, Debbie punched her brother when he reached for the remote control to change the television channel.

Siblings need to get the message that the feelings they experience (anger, jealousy, resentment, etc.) are normal and acceptable, but that misbehavior in expressing those feelings is not acceptable. After about a week of Debbie stomping around, generally mistreating family members, and being sent to her room and grounded repeatedly, her mother, Anne, decided enough was enough. On a Saturday morning, Anne arranged for her husband to spend the morning with Jason while she took Debbie shopping. After a relaxing morning, Anne and Debbie had lunch together. Over lunch, Anne asked Debbie about her behavior. Debbie, very matter-of-factly, said, "Jason gets away with it. Besides, no one ever pays attention to me." Anne and Debbie agreed that they would make having lunch together once each month a priority and that Debbie would start spending some extra time with her favorite aunt. In addition, they talked about Debbie's feelings. Anne told Debbie that it is OK to feel angry and jealous but that she still has to act appropriately. Anne made it clear that there would always be consequences for negative behavior. Anne also talked with Jason's therapist and made arrangements for Debbie to meet with her so that Debbie could gain a better understanding of how Jason's symptoms affect his behavior.

Siblings can benefit greatly from participation in family therapy or short-term individual therapy aimed at increasing understanding and building coping skills related to their sibling's mood disorder.

WITHDRAWAL

Whereas some siblings act out, others pull away and withdraw from the family. Some may withdraw altogether, and others may move toward friends and school. For adolescents, moving away from family and toward peers is an expected and important part of development. The key here is that your teenager is not pulling away too much or too soon because she does not feel valued or supported at home.

Nine-year old Dave is sick and tired of being cautious not to set off his brother, Nick. As a result, Dave started spending more and more time in his room. He never asked his mother to take him places, because he didn't want to bother her. Instead, he took every opportunity to spend time with neighborhood friends so he could be out of the house. Dave's father, Ken, began to notice that Dave was in his room more and more. One evening, Ken knocked on Dave's door. As Ken started to ask Dave how things were going, Dave became tearful and described his frustration and loneliness. The first thing Ken did was to assure Dave that protecting his mother was not his job. Then they started a list of things Ken and Dave could do together to make life better for Dave. This list included joining some recreational activities, including Boy Scouts and an after-school chess club. Following that discussion, Dave's parents decided that it was important to address Nick's ongoing irritability with his treatment team, as it clearly was interfering with their home life.

MAINTAINING SAFETY

In some cases the safety of siblings becomes an issue. Siblings of children with bipolar disorder are often the targets of aggression. At times they may fear getting hurt or may worry that their personal property will be destroyed. Some helpful strategies include installing locks on bedroom doors (with the parents always being able to access the key for safety), providing lock boxes or other secure places for important belongings, and helping siblings develop plans concerning where they will go and what they will do when they are feeling particularly vulnerable. Siblings need to know that parents are aware of and concerned about their safety, whether the risk is physical or emotional.

At times Debbie was terrified of Jason. She feared that he would hurt her but also found his screaming incredibly stressful. Eventually Debbie told her parents that she wanted to have a place she could go where it would be quiet and she could feel safe. They had already put a lock on her bedroom door but decided to add a lock to her closet door.

They added some pillows, a small radio, a lamp, and a couple of posters to her closet walls and made a reading nook where she could retreat whenever she needed.

SOCIAL ISOLATION

Siblings of children with mood disorders can become isolated for a variety of reasons:

- Avoiding having friends over due to embarrassment
- Avoiding talking about family life as a result of stigma
- Not asking to participate in activities to avoid being a "burden"

Regardless of the reason, siblings can end up having limited peer networks and being underinvolved in activities. Parents can help by providing safe ways to have friends over (e.g., supervising closely; timing visits to coincide with the sibling's visit to Grandma) and by making sure that siblings are involved in some activities outside the home.

Trisha is fourteen and has a younger brother, Scott, with bipolar disorder. Last time she had a friend over, a year ago, her brother gave her friend a bear hug and grabbed her breast. Since then, Trisha had not asked any of her friends to come over. Her friends talk constantly about their problems at home. Trisha is sure that if she talked about her brother her friends would think she was a freak. So she listens quietly and says little. As Scott began doing better (an atypical antipsychotic was added to his regimen, and his mood stabilized significantly), Trisha's parents began to notice that she was spending a lot of time away from the family. When they asked her how things were going, she shrugged. Trisha explained her fears about having friends over. Despite Scott's significant improvement, he still tended to be hyperactive and to intrude in conversations inappropriately. Trisha's parents were concerned about Trisha's experiences. They talked about how Trisha could get together with her friends. They decided that letting Trisha organize outings (to the mall, movies, ice skating rink, etc.) for which her parents would provide the transportation was the best solution.

Define Sibling Roles

It's natural for healthy siblings to take on roles in the family, such as "the healthy child," "the peacemaker," and "the protector." Siblings need support and assistance from parents to figure out what their roles should be and to avoid taking on "jobs" that they shouldn't assume. The only role a sibling should be encouraged to take on in the family is that of a healthy child, growing up and addressing his or her own developmental needs. This is enough to keep any child or teenager busy!

Communicate

Keeping channels of communication open is critical with siblings. Talk to them periodically. Listen without correcting. Give feedback, but stay positive. Return to our discussion of communication in Chapter 8 and rethink how it applies to the siblings in your family.

Being the sibling of a child or teen with a mood disorder can be stressful for many reasons. Families have limited time and financial resources, and siblings often suffer because their needs are less pressing. Sibling challenges can be short term and acute (how to stay safe from aggressive behavior, for one) or longer term and chronic (e.g., How do you manage the stress of living with someone who is frequently irritable and doesn't hesitate to take it out on you?). As a parent, you can help siblings by recognizing their feelings; talking with them frequently; helping them get a caring, listening ear outside the home; connecting them to healthy activities; obtaining, if needed, appropriate treatment for them; and, most of all, taking care of yourself so that you can be the best possible parent to all your children.

14 How to Take Care of Yourself

As the parent of a child or teenager with a mood disorder, you can end up beleaguered by the demands of the job. You may become so wrapped up in efforts to help your son or daughter, to manage the child's behavior and to keep peace at home, and to foster a normal, healthy family life that you hardly notice when you're not feeling well yourself, when you're exhausted, or when your reserves of energy and hope are dangerously close to empty. This chapter is for you and only you. Not for you as treatment monitor, behavior management specialist, damage control artist, or head of household, but for you as an individual who needs care and support as much as your mood-impaired child and the rest of your family do. You need to take care of yourself—not just when you finally have a little spare time but especially when you have none at all. After all, you can't take care of anyone or anything else if you've exhausted your own resources.

Many parents we know have described to us those awful moments when they finally pause to take a deep breath in the middle of a hectic day and realize they feel not only wiped out but achingly alone in their struggles. We hope that by now you realize you're not alone, that many families struggle with the same issues you've been facing. Parents *routinely* experience guilt, powerlessness, denial, anger (at themselves, the other parent, their parents, the school, the psychiatrist, the world, God, the person driving in front of them, etc.), anxiety, fear, uncertainty, confusion, blame, and shame. Through this book we hope to help you:

- Let go of guilt
- Become empowered

- Accept the reality and begin to take action
- Channel your anger productively
- Gain tools to relieve your anxiety and fear
- Eliminate some uncertainty and accept what is unavoidable
- Become less confused
- Stop blaming (yourself and others)
- Overcome shame and stigma

Read through the rest of this chapter, review the previous chapters, then reread this list to see how you can apply our recommendations to reaching these goals.

Combating Isolation

One of the biggest dangers of parenthood is isolation. Almost any problem can seem insurmountable if you have no help or support. Parents of children with mood disorders have, if anything, a greater need for practical assistance and emotional support, yet having a child with a mental illness makes isolation more likely. Embarrassment about your child's behavior, hurt caused by "helpful" comments about how better discipline could "solve" the problem, and general exhaustion all contribute to keeping you apart from friends, relatives, and supportive comrades in the battle against mood disorders. Maybe you feel you just don't have a moment to get together with the people who can lend a sympathetic ear or make you laugh or just make you feel better when they're nearby. Or maybe you have a large network of friends and/or family living nearby but no one you can comfortably confide in and count on to help you when you most need assistance. Isolation can be real or perceived. Either way, it's an additional drain on your already depleted strength.

So where do you start? Think about who is in your current network. Can you reach out to anyone who might become a resource for you? Are there ways that you can build your network? Have you contacted community agencies to find parent support groups? Do you belong to a church, synagogue, or mosque through which you can access support? Can you access online support? Most important, don't accept isolation as the only possibility. Take action. Reach out to others in similar need and become a support for one another.

Meeting Your Needs

If you're like most parents of children with mood disorders, you may never even think about your own needs. Not surprisingly, your child's needs tend to come first. But it is important that you also attend to your own needs. As we've said before, this is a marathon, not a sprint. You need to sustain your own mood and energy level in order to have positive energy to deal with your child or teenager who has a mood disorder.

Respite Care

Every parent needs opportunities for a break—time to go for a walk or a jog (more on exercise later), nap, run errands, read a book, or spend time with friends or with his or her other children. Respite care provides this—a break or a rest. Respite can be provided informally through arrangements with friends or family members or formally through agencies. Depending on where you live, access to respite may be limited. If you don't have access to respite through friends or family members, ask your treatment team members or contact local agencies. Depending on your situation and available resources, respite care may involve someone taking your child to do an activity for a couple of hours or could involve your child spending a night or weekend away from home. Respite care should be set up to meet your needs, with your child's needs in mind.

Share Parenting Duties

Some parenting tasks are easy or fun, whereas others can be frustrating and difficult (setting limits with an irritable and depressed adolescent is trying; getting a child dressed who wakes up grumpy and doesn't want to go to school can be maddening). So divide and conquer, or share the pain.

Preserve Couple Time

Raising a child with special needs (and a mood disorder certainly qualifies for this distinction) can be very hard on a relationship. In addition to the potential for disagreements about treatment and management issues, time is a valuable commodity. Don't neglect your relationship in the name of caring for your children. Your spouse or parenting partner is an important source of support and assistance. Take care of that relationship. Make time to spend alone together. Schedule dates—even if you have them in your family room with a rented movie! If you're in conflict about your child's treatment, seek parent guidance to help you get on the same track. If you have conflicts that you are unable to work out, seek couples therapy. Your personal and intimate relationships are part of what keeps you healthy and happy. When you're healthy and happy, you're a better parent.

Gabe had been raising his son and daughter (now thirteen and ten) alone since his wife had passed away seven years ago. He had worked hard to help his daughter get the right treatment and learn good coping skills for managing depression and anxiety. Sarah had been taking medication and working with the same therapist since she was seven. Sarah's therapist had also provided support and guidance to Gabe. When Gabe met Margaret, he wasn't sure how far to let the relationship go. He hesitated before introducing his children to Margaret but in the end decided to go ahead. As he and Margaret got closer and she began to develop relationships with Sarah and Jeremy, he brought the subject of his relationship with Margaret to the therapist. The therapist had been supportive of Gabe's relationship with Margaret from the beginning, and when Gabe brought up the topic of marrying Margaret, she cheered. She told Gabe that she had observed only positive changes since Margaret had come into their lives. Sarah was benefiting from having a close relationship with a woman, as was Jeremy. And Gabe clearly seemed happier and less stressed. The therapist told Gabe that she thought marriage would only solidify and strengthen an already good thing (although there is always some adjustment when a parent remarries).

Becoming a Good Stress Manager

The first step in becoming a good manager of stress is to make a realistic assessment of how much stress you can handle and still remain healthy yourself. Some people thrive on constant activity, whereas others need a large dose of peace and quiet each day. There is no right or wrong to any of these patterns. The important thing is to know yourself and to do what you can to match your world to your temperament.

So take some time to think through where you fit on the continuum. If you have too much stress in your life, can you find ways to simplify?

There is no particular formula for how best to do this. It depends on your lifestyle and needs. Following are a few ideas to get you going. Just remember, deciding what should stay and what should go is up to you!

- Explore changes to your and/or your spouse's work schedule. Can you
  —reduce your hours?
  —work flexible hours?
  - go in a little earlier to come home earlier?
  - go in later to make mornings less chaotic?
  - work four longer days to have one weekday off?
- Delegate household tasks.
- Examine your children's schedules—are they too full?
- Prioritize your "to do" list. Can some items on the bottom of the list be eliminated?

Free Medicine

The most important part of managing stress is taking good care of yourself. We like to call the list of health behaviors we discuss here "free medicine." By this we mean that these behaviors don't cost money and have no bad side effects and that studies have proven them to be good for your mental health!

- Practice good sleep habits.
  —Get enough sleep.
  —Go to bed and get up at the same time each day.
- Eat healthfully.
  —Eat a well-balanced diet.
  —Snack on nutritious foods.
  This benefits the entire family. Not only will you be healthier, but your children will have better food choices available to them. This helps both to curb hunger-induced irritability and to counteract weight gain from medications.
- Exercise regularly.
  —Research has shown the benefit of regular exercise for mood and general mental health.
  —Find fun ways to exercise that involve your family or use your exercise time as "me" time.

- Plan fun activities for your family.
- Maintain your support system.

    Earlier in the chapter we wrote about building your support network. Once you have a support network, be sure to maintain it. Invite a friend for a cup of coffee or go to a movie with your sister.
- Write in a journal.

    Studies have shown the beneficial effects of writing as a way to "unload" negative feelings and to gain perspective on problems.
- Recognize the role of spirituality in your life.

    —Make prayer, meditation, or a time to think quietly part of your daily routine.

    —Participate in organized religion if this is a comfortable part of your tradition. A faith-based community can provide support on a variety of levels for families with special needs.
- Keep your sense of humor—laughing helps you:

    —Relieve tension.

    —Diffuse a difficult interaction with your child or teen.

Remain Hopeful

It's unlikely that you will exhaust every possible treatment option (especially because new options are becoming available all the time). Allow bad days just to be bad days and not the new reality. Use your mental health team and support network as your sounding boards. Keep in mind that new treatments are being developed as you read.

Avoid Martyrdom

To be the best parent you can be, you will have to be good to yourself. Don't martyr yourself—your children need you! Tanya realized she was at the end of her rope when one day, while driving back to school to pick up her son's math book, she alternated between screaming and crying the whole way to school and back. Tanya had been working so very hard to hold it all together. As a single mom, she had managed to figure out that Will had a significant problem. She got him a good evaluation and treatment and began attending family therapy sessions with him every other week. Tanya managed to rearrange her hours at work so that she could do this without getting docked pay, as they would never be able to pay their existing and new bills (therapy co-payments, medication costs, and a membership at the local health club where Tanya, Will, and his sister Tracy could enjoy some active time together) if her paycheck shrank. And now Will had just informed her that he was failing algebra and that if he didn't have his book to study for Friday's test he'd get an F for the quarter.

Tanya thought long and hard that evening. The depth of her anger and frustration scared her. If she couldn't manage to cope with her family's situation she didn't know what she would do. But, she knew for certain that things couldn't go on the way they had been. The next night, Tanya rented a movie for Will and Tracy, popped them some popcorn, then gave them strict orders to stay in the family room and leave her alone for the next two hours. She drew a nice, hot bath, poured herself a refreshing cool drink, and sank into the bubbles. An hour later, when every muscle in her body had unwound, she got out of the tub and began to write in her journal. Tanya used to keep a journal as a college student but hadn't written an entry in the past twenty years. Tanya began by outlining all of her responsibilities. Next, she drew five columns on a second sheet of paper. She labeled these *Tanya, Will, Tracy, Roger* (her ex-husband), and *Other*. She then started rewriting her list of responsibilities, but this time into the five columns, until every column had one or more entries. Tanya rehearsed the conversations she would have tomorrow with Will, Tracy, Roger, and her mother, who had been allocated several tasks in the "other" column. She called downstairs to the kids to tell them it was time for bed and resolved to have a family meeting in the morning to review the new plans. Tanya fell asleep peacefully that night, more relaxed than she had felt in months.

Recognize Negative Feelings

Recognize and accept that you're likely to feel resentful or angry sometimes. You may feel resentful that your spouse "gets" to go to work all day while you deal with the challenges of raising your child. You may feel angry or tired or just plain sick of the daily challenges. Accept your feelings. It takes far more emotional energy to pretend those feelings aren't there than it does to acknowledge them and then make a plan to deal with them. Gain perspective by journaling and/or openly discussing your feelings with your spouse, your therapist, or someone else in your support network.

Minimize the Impact

If and when you are in a crisis mode, it will probably be impossible for you not to feel as if your child's condition has "taken over" family life. However, once you're out of crisis mode, do your best to turn your attention to the needs of all family members. Attend to the cares and concerns of the "three S's"—siblings, spouse, and self—in addition to your child and his symptoms.

Grieving

During pregnancy or while awaiting the adoption of a child, you might have daydreamed about what your child would be like. What would she like to do? What would he be good at? What will she be when she grows up? What will he look like? No one thinks, "I wonder what medication combination my child will need?" or "How will I juggle going to two mental health visits per week for a year?"

The grief parents experience when they realize that their child has a lifelong, biologically based illness is real. The healthy child you had hoped and planned for needs regular therapy and daily medication. At each developmental phase (e.g., transitions to middle school and high school; graduation), you will experience reminders about how your child is different. Give yourself time and permission to grieve and grieve again each time your child makes a developmental shift.

In Closing

In this chapter we have emphasized the importance of taking care of yourself. We have referred several times to thinking about your life as a marathon, not a sprint. Running a marathon involves good coaching, good conditioning, and a good attitude. Don't hesitate to seek help for yourself if you need it to optimize your ability to function as a parent. Take care of yourself, both mentally and physically. This can only help you and your child. Remain hopeful. Investing in yourself and your child *will* make a difference.

Resources

Books

Depression

FOR CHILDREN

Dubuque, N., & Dubuque, S. (1996). *Kid power tactics for dealing with depression.* King of Prussia, PA: Center for Applied Psychology.

FOR ADOLESCENTS

Cobain, B. (1998). *When nothing matters anymore: A survival guide for depressed teens.* Minneapolis, MN: Free Spirit.

Copeland, M. E., & Copans, S. (2002) *Recovering from depression: A workbook for teens.* Baltimore: Brookes.

Irwin, C. (1999). *Conquering the beast within: How I fought depression and won . . . and how you can too.* New York: Random House.

Koplewicz, H. S. (2002) *More than moody: Recognizing and treating adolescent depression.* New York: Putnam Press.

FOR PARENTS

Dubuque, S. (1996). *A parent's survival guide to childhood depression.* King of Prussia, PA: Center for Applied Psychology.

Seligman, M. E. P. (1996). *The optimistic child.* New York: HarperCollins Publishers.

FOR ADULTS

Beardslee, W. (2002). *Out of the darkened room: Protecting the children and strengthening the family when a parent is depressed.* Boston: Little, Brown.

Copeland, M. E. (2001). *Living without depression and manic depression.* Oakland, CA: New Harbinger.

Greenberger, D., & Padesky, C. A. (1995). *Mind over mood.* New York: Guilford Press.

Whybrow, P. *A mood apart.* New York: HarperCollins Publishers.

Bipolar Disorder

FOR CHILDREN

Child and Adolescent Bipolar Foundation (CABF) and Depression and Bipolar Support Alliance. (2003). *The storm in my brain.* Wilmette, IL: CABF.

McGee, C. (2002). *Matt the moody hermit crab.* Nashville, TN: McGee & Woods.

FOR ADOLESCENTS

Summers, M. A. (2000). *Everything you need to know about bipolar disorder and manic depressive illness.* New York: Rosen.

FOR YOUNG ADULTS

Simon, L. (2002). *Detour.* New York: Simon & Schuster.

FOR PARENTS

Findling, R. L., Kowatch, R. A., & Post, R. M. (2003). *Pediatric bipolar disorder: A handbook for clinicians.* London: Martin Dunitz.

Geller, B., & Del Bello, M. P. (Eds.). (2003). *Bipolar disorder in childhood and early adolescence.* New York: Guilford Press.

Papalos, D., & Papalos, J. (2002) *The bipolar child.* New York: Broadway Books.

Waltz, M. (2000). *Bipolar disorders: A guide to helping children and adolescents.* Sebastopol, CA: O'Reilly & Associates.

FOR ADULTS

Hinshaw, S. P. (2002). *The years of silence are past: My father's life with bipolar disorder.* Cambridge, UK: Cambridge University Press.

Jamison, J. R. (1995). *An unquiet mind.* New York: Knopf.

Miklowitz, D. J. (2002). *The bipolar disorder survival guide.* New York: Guilford Press.

Parenting Issues

Faber, A., & Mazlish, E. (1998). *Siblings without rivalry.* New York: Avon Books.

Faber, A., & Mazlish, E. (1999). *How to talk so kids will listen and listen so kids will talk.* New York: Avon Books.

Reivich, K., & Shatte, A. (2002). *The resilience factor: 7 essential skills for overcoming life's inevitable obstacles.* New York: Random House.

Psychiatric Disorders

Faraone, S. V. (2003). *Straight talk about your child's mental health.* New York: Guilford Press.

Greene, R. (1998). *The explosive child.* New York: HarperCollins.

Koplewicz, H. (1996). *It's nobody's fault.* New York: Times Books.

Medication

Wilens, T. E. (2001). *Straight talk about psychiatric medications for kids* (rev. ed.). New York: Guilford Press.

Complementary Interventions

Seasonal Affective Disorder

Light Boxes
www.nmha.org/infoctr/factsheets/27.cfm

Rosenthal, N. E. (1998). *Winter blues.* New York: Guilford Press.

Nutritional Interventions

EMpowerplus
1-888-878-3467
www.truehope.com

Omega-3 Fatty Acids
1-800-383-2030
www.omegabrite.com

Side Effect Management

Bedwetting
DRI Sleeper
1-877 331 2768
www.dri-sleeper.com

General Information
1-800-214-9605
www.bedwettingstore.com

Weight Management
Information about children's mental and physical health
via separate areas for children, adolescents, and parents
www.kidshealth.org

National Organizations

Child and Adolescent Bipolar Foundation (CABF)
1-847-256-8525
www.bpkids.org

Depression and Bipolar Support Alliance (DBSA)
1-800-826-3632
dbsalliance.org

Juvenile Bipolar Research Foundation (JBRF)
www.jbrf.org

National Alliance for the Mentally Ill (NAMI)
1-800-950-6264
www.nami.org

National Mental Health Association (NMHA)
1-703-684-7722
www.nmha.org

School Planning

Child and Adolescent Bipolar Foundation
www.cabf.org/learning

Packer, L. E. *Classroom Tips for Children with Bipolar Disorder*
www.schoolbehavior.com

Parent information and school planning ideas for children
and adolescents with depression
www.redflags.org

State Boards of Education
www.nasbe.org/SEA_Links/SEA_Links.html

Therapeutic Boarding Schools: The National Association
of Therapeutic Schools and Programs (NATSAP)
www.natsap.org

U.S. Department of Education
www.ed.gov/index.jsp
www.ed.gov/pubs/edpubs.html

Wright, P. W. D., & Wright, P. D. (2002). *From emotions to advocacy: The special education survival guide.* Hartfield, VA: Harbor House Law Press.
www.wrightslaw.com

Governmental Supplemental Security Income

www.ssa.gov/notices/supplemental-security-income

Comorbid Conditions

Attention-Deficit/Hyperactivity Disorder

Barkley, R. A. (2000). *Taking charge of ADHD.* New York: Guilford Press.
Parker, H. C. (1999). *Put yourself in their shoes: Understanding teenagers with attention deficit hyperactivity disorder.* Plantation, FL: Specialty Press.

Oppositional Defiant Disorder

Barkley, R. A., & Benton, C. M. (1998). *Your defiant child: Eight steps to better behavior.* New York: Guilford Press.

Anxiety Disorders

Rapee, R., Spence, S., Cobham, V., & Wignall, A. (2000). *Helping your anxious child.* Oakland, CA: New Harbinger.

Obsessive–Compulsive Disorder

Chansky, T. E. (2000). *Freeing your child from obsessive–compulsive disorder.* New York: Crown.
Waltz, M. (2000). *Obsessive–compulsive disorder: Help for children and adolescents.* Sebastopol, CA: O'Reilly & Assoc.

Eating Disorders

Pipher, M. (1995). *Hunger pains: The modern woman's tragic quest for thinness.* New York: Ballantine Books.

Asperger Syndrome

Ozonoff, S., Dawson, G., & McPartland, J. (2002) *A parents' guide to Asperger syndrome and high-functioning autism.* New York: Guilford Press.

References

Chapter 1

Findling, R. L., Kowatch, R. A., & Post, R. M. (2003). *Pediatric bipolar disorder: A handbook for clinicians.* London: Martin Dunitz.

Lewinsohn, P. M., Klein, D. N., & Seeley, J. R. (1995). Bipolar disorders in a community sample of older adolescents: Prevalence, phenomenology, comorbidity, and course. *Journal of the American Academy of Child and Adolescent Psychiatry, 34*(4), 454–463.

Weissman, M. M., Bland, R. C., Canino, G. J., Faravelli, C., Greenwald, S., Hwu, H. G., et al. (1996). Cross-national epidemiology of major depression and bipolar disorder. *Journal of the American Medical Association, 276*(4), 293–299.

Wozniak, J., Biederman, J., Kiely, K., Ablon, J. S., Faraone, S. V., Mundy, E., & Mennin, D. (1995). Mania-like symptoms suggestive of childhood-onset bipolar disorder in clinically referred children. *Journal of the American Academy of Child and Adolescent Psychiatry, 34*(7), 867–876.

Chapter 2

Fristad, M. A., Gavazzi, S. M., & Soldano, K. W. (1999). Naming the enemy: Learning to differentiate the "symptoms" from the "self" that experiences them. *Journal of Family Psychotherapy, 10*(1), 81–88.

Geller, B., Bolhofner, K., Craney, J. L., Williams, M., DelBello, M. P., & Gundersen, K. (2000). Psychosocial functioning in a prepubertal and early adolescent bipolar disorder phenotype. *Journal of the American Academy of Child and Adolescent Psychiatry, 39*(12), 1543–1548.

Geller, B., Zimerman, B., Williams, M., DelBello, M., Bolhofner, K., Craney, J. L., Frazier, J., et al. (2002a). DSM-IV mania symptoms in a prepubertal and early adolescent bipolar disorder phenotype compared to attention-deficit hyperactive and normal controls. *Journal of Child and Adolescent Psychopharmacology, 12*(1), 11–25.

Geller, B., Zimerman, B., Williams, M., DelBello, M., Frazier, J., & Beringer, L. (2002b). Phenomenology of prepubertal and early adolescent bipolar disorder: Examples of elated mood, grandiose behaviors, decreased need for sleep, racing thoughts and hypersexuality. *Journal of Child and Adolescent Psychopharmacology, 12*(1), 3–9.

Kovacs, M., Akiskal, H. S., Gatsonis, C., & Parrone, P. L. (1994). Childhood-onset dysthymic disorder. Clinical features and prospective naturalistic outcome. *Archives of General Psychiatry, 51,* 365–374.

Chapter 3

Birmaher, B., Ryan, N. D., Williamson, D. E., Brent, D. A., Kaufman, J., Dahl, R. E., et al. (1996). Childhood and adolescent depression: A review of the past 10 years (Part I). *Journal of the American Academy of Child and Adolescent Psychiatry, 35*(1), 1427–1439.

Gershon, E. S., Hamovit, J. H., Guroff, J., & Nurnberger, J. I. (1987). Birth-cohort changes in manic and depressive disorders in relatives of bipolar and schizoaffective patients. *Archives of General Psychiatry, 44,* 314–319.

Lange, K. J., & McInnis, M. G. (2002). Studies of anticipation in bipolar affective disorder. *CNS Spectrum, 7,* 196–202.

Mendlewicz, J., Lindbald, K., Souery, D., Mahieu, B., Nylander, P. O., Bruyn, A. D., et al. (1997). Expanded trinucleotide CAG repeats in families with bipolar affective disorder. *Biological Psychiatry, 42,* 1115–1122.

Chapter 4

American Psychiatric Association (1994). *Diagnostic and statistical manual of mental disorders* (4th ed.). Washington, DC: Author.

Carlson, G. A. (1996). Clinical features and pathogenesis of child and adolescent mania. In K. I. Shulman, M. Tohen, & S. P. Kutcher (Eds.), *Mood disorders across the lifespan* (pp. 127–147). New York: Wiley-Liss.

Findling, R. L., Gracious, B. L., McNamara, N. K., Youngstrom, E. A., Demeter, C. A., Branicky, L. A., & Calabrese, J. R. (2001). Rapid continuous cycling and psychiatric co-morbidity in pediatric bipolar I disorder. *Bipolar Disorders, 3,* 202–210.

Geller, B., & Luby, J. (1997). Child and adolescent bipolar disorder: A review of the past 10 years. *Journal of the American Academy of Child and Adolescent Psychiatry, 36*(9), 1168–1176.

Geller, B., Zimerman, B., Williams, M., DelBello, M., Bolhofner, K., Craney, J. L., et al. (2002). DSM-IV mania symptoms in a prepubertal and early adolescent bipolar disorder phenotype compared to attention-deficit hyperactive and normal controls. *Journal of Child and Adolescent Psychopharmacology, 12*(1), 11–25.

Lagace, D. C., Kutcher, S. P., & Robertson, H. A. (2003). Mathematics deficits in adolescents with bipolar I disorder. *American Journal of Psychiatry, 160*(1), 100–104.

Wozniak, J., Biederman, J., Kiely, K., Ablon, J. S., Faraone, S. V., Mundy, E., et al. (1995). Mania-like symptoms suggestive of childhood-onset bipolar disorder in clinically referred children. *Journal of the American Academy of Child and Adolescent Psychiatry, 34*(7), 867–876.

Chapter 5

Kaplan, B. J., Crawford, S. G., Gardner, B., & Farrelly, G. (2002). Treatment of mood lability and explosive rage with mineral and vitamins: Two case studies in children. *Journal of Child and Adolescent Psychopharmacology, 12*(3), 205–219.

Kaplan, B. J., Simpson, J. S. A., Ferre, R. C., Gorman, C. P., McMullen, D. M., & Crawford, S. G. (2001). Effective mood stabilization with a chelated mineral supplement: An open-label trial in bipolar disorder. *Journal of Clinical Psychiatry, 62*(12), 936–944.

Nemets, B., Stahl, Z., & Belmaker, R. H. (2002). Addition of omega-3 fatty acid to maintenance medication treatment for recurrent unipolar depressive disorder. *American Journal of Psychiatry, 159*, 477–479.

Stoll, A. L., Severus, W. E., Freeman, M. P., Rueter, S., Zboyan, H. A., Diamond, E., et al. (1999). Omega 3 fatty acids in bipolar disorder. A preliminary double-blind placebo-controlled study. *Archives of General Psychiatry, 56*, 407–412.

Swedo, S. E., Allen, J. A., Glod, C. A., Clark, C. H., Techer, M. H., Richter, D., et al. (1997). A controlled study of light therapy for the treatment of pediatric seasonal affective disorder. *Journal of the American Academy of Child and Adolescent Psychiatry, 36*(6), 816–821.

Chapter 6

Chiaie, R. D., Pancheri, P., & Scapicchio, P. (2002). Efficacy and tolerability of oral and intramuscular S-adenosyl-L-methione 1, 4-butanedisulfonate (SAMe) in the treatment of major depression: Comparison with imipramine in 2 multicenter studies. *American Journal of Clinical Nutrition, 76*(5), 1172S–1176S.

Findling, R. L., McNamara, N. K., O'Riordan, M. A., Reed, M. D., DeMeter, C. A., Branicky, L. A., & Blumer, J. L. (2003). An open-label pilot study of St. John's Wort in juvenile depression. *Journal of the American Academy of Child and Adolescent Psychiatry, 42*(8), 908–914.

Frazier, J. A., Meyer, M. C., Biederman, J., Wozniak, J., Wilens, T. E., Spencer, T. J., et al. (1999). Risperidone treatment for juvenile bipolar disorder: A retrospective chart review. *Journal of the American Academy of Child and Adolescent Psychiatry, 38*(8), 960–965.

Jurgens, T. M. (1999). The use of herbal medicines in younger psychiatric patients. *Child and Adolescent Psychopharmacology News, 4*, 2–4.

Linde, K., Ramierz, G., Muldrow, C. D., Pauls, A., Weidenhammer, W., & Melchart, D. (1996). St. John's wort for depression: An overview and meta-analysis of randomised clinical trials. *British Medical Journal, 313*, 253–258.

Wilens, T. E. (2001). *Straight talk about psychiatric medications for kids.* New York: Guilford Press.

Chapter 7

Brent, D. A., Poling, K., McKain, B., & Baugher, M. (1993). A psychoeducational program for families of affectively ill children and adolescents. *Journal of the American Academy for Child and Adolescent Psychiatry, 32*(4), 770–774.

Fristad, M. A., Goldberg-Arnold, J. S., & Gavazzi, S. M. (2002). Multifamily psychoeducation groups (MFPG) for families of children with bipolar disorder. *Bipolar Disorders, 4*, 254–262.

Kaslow, N. J., & Racusin, G. R. (1994). Family therapy for depression in young people. In W. M. Reynolds & H. F. Johnston (Eds.), *Handbook of depression in children and adolescents* (pp. 345–363). New York: Plenum Press.

Marcotte, D. (1997). Treating depression in adolescence: A review of the effectiveness of cognitive-behavioral treatments. *Journal of Youth and Adolescence, 26*(3), 149–154.

Mufson, L., & Fairbanks, J. (1996). Interpersonal therapy for depressed adolescents: A one-year naturalistic follow-up study. *Journal of the American Academy of Child and Adolescent Psychiatry, 35*(9), 1145–1155.

Reinecke, M. A., Ryan, N. E., & DuBois, D. L. (1998). Cognitive-behavioral therapy of depression and depressive symptoms during adolescence: A review and meta-analysis. *Journal of the American Academy of Child and Adolescent Psychiatry, 37*(1), 26–34.

Stark, K. D., Reynolds, W. M., & Kaslow, N. J. (1987). A comparison of the relative efficacy of self-control therapy and a behavioral problem-solving therapy for depression in children. *Journal of Abnormal Child Psychology, 15*(1), 91–113.

Stark, K. D., Swearer, S., Kurowski, C., Sommer, D., & Bowen, B. (1996). Targeting the child and the family: A holistic approach to treating child and adolescent depressive disorders. In E. D. Hibbs & P. S. Jensen (Eds.), *Psychosocial treatments for child and adolescent disorders: Empirically based strategies for clinical practice* (pp. 207–238). Washington, DC: American Psychological Association.

Weisz, J. R., Thurber, C. A., Sweeney, L., Proffitt, V. D., & LeGagnoux, G. L. (1997). Brief treatment of mild-to-moderate child depression using primary and secondary control enhancement training. *Journal of Consulting and Clinical Psychology, 65*(4), 703–707.

Wood, A., Harrington, R., & Moore, A. (1996). Controlled trial of a brief cognitive-behavioural intervention in adolescent patients with depressive disorders. *Journal of Child Psychology and Psychiatry and Allied Disciplines, 37*(6), 737–746

Chapter 9

Goldberg-Arnold, J. S., & Fristad, M. A. (2003). Psychotherapy for children with bipolar disorder. In B. Geller & M. Del Bello (Eds.), *Bipolar disorder in childhood and early adolescence.* New York: Guilford Press.

Chapter 10

The educational needs of a child or adolescent with bipolar disorder. Retrieved May 24, 2003, from www.bpkids.org/learning/educating.htm.

Chapter 11

Kann, L., Kinchen, S. A., Williams, B. I., Ross, J. G., Lowry, R., Hill, C. V., et al. (1998, August 14). *Youth Risk Behavior Surveillance—United States, 1997* (CDC Surveillance Surveys, Vol. 47, No. SS-3). Atlanta, GA: Centers for Disease Control.

Chapter 12

Holder, D., & Anderson, C. M. (1990). Psychoeducational family intervention for depressed patients and their families. In G. I. Keitner (Ed.), *Depression and families: Impact and treatment* (pp. 157–184). Washington, DC: American Psychiatric Press.

Chapter 14

Esterling, B. A., L'Abate, L., Murray, E. J., & Pennebaker, J. W. (1999). Empirical foundations for writing in prevention and psychotherapy: Mental and physical health outcomes. *Clinical Psychology Review, 19*(1), 79–96.

Index

About the Authors

Mary A. Fristad, PhD, ABPP, is Professor of Psychiatry and Psychology at the Ohio State University and the Director of Research and Psychological Services in the OSU Division of Child and Adolescent Psychiatry. Her area of specialty is childhood mood disorders. She has published more than 100 articles and book chapters addressing the assessment and treatment of childhood-onset depression, suicidality, and bipolar disorder, and recently coedited the *Handbook of Serious Emotional Disturbance in Children and Adolescents* (John Wiley & Sons). Dr. Fristad has been the principal or co-principal investigator on over a dozen federal, state, local, and industry grants. Currently, she is conducting a five-year National Institute of Mental Health grant to investigate the efficacy of multifamily psychoeducation groups in treating childhood mood disorders and a two-year Ohio Department of Mental Health grant to investigate the efficacy of individual family psychoeducation in treating early-onset bipolar disorder in children.

Jill S. Goldberg Arnold, PhD, did her graduate work at the State University of New York at Binghamton and completed her postdoctoral training at the Ohio State University. She then joined the Division of Child and Adolescent Psychiatry at OSU, where she was Clinical Assistant Professor of Psychiatry and specialized in childhood mood disorders. She has collaborated on both state and federally funded research projects examining the impact of multifamily psychoeducation for families of children with mood disorders. Dr. Goldberg Arnold has multiple publications in the area of childhood mood disorders. Currently, Dr. Goldberg Arnold has a private practice in Bryn Mawr, Pennsylvania.